Cognitive Psychodynamics as an Integrative Framework in Counselling Psychology and Psychotherapy

AF166378

Tony Ward · Arnaud Plagnol

Cognitive Psychodynamics as an Integrative Framework in Counselling Psychology and Psychotherapy

palgrave
macmillan

Tony Ward
Department of Health and Social Sciences
University of the West of England
Bristol, UK

Arnaud Plagnol
Paris 8 University
St. Denis, France

ISBN 978-3-030-25825-2   ISBN 978-3-030-25823-8   (eBook)
https://doi.org/10.1007/978-3-030-25823-8

© The Editor(s) (if applicable) and The Author(s) 2019
This work is subject to copyright. All rights are solely and exclusively licensed by the Publisher, whether the whole or part of the material is concerned, specifically the rights of translation, reprinting, reuse of illustrations, recitation, broadcasting, reproduction on microfilms or in any other physical way, and transmission or information storage and retrieval, electronic adaptation, computer software, or by similar or dissimilar methodology now known or hereafter developed.
The use of general descriptive names, registered names, trademarks, service marks, etc. in this publication does not imply, even in the absence of a specific statement, that such names are exempt from the relevant protective laws and regulations and therefore free for general use.
The publisher, the authors and the editors are safe to assume that the advice and information in this book are believed to be true and accurate at the date of publication. Neither the publisher nor the authors or the editors give a warranty, expressed or implied, with respect to the material contained herein or for any errors or omissions that may have been made. The publisher remains neutral with regard to jurisdictional claims in published maps and institutional affiliations.

This Palgrave Macmillan imprint is published by the registered company Springer Nature Switzerland AG
The registered company address is: Gewerbestrasse 11, 6330 Cham, Switzerland

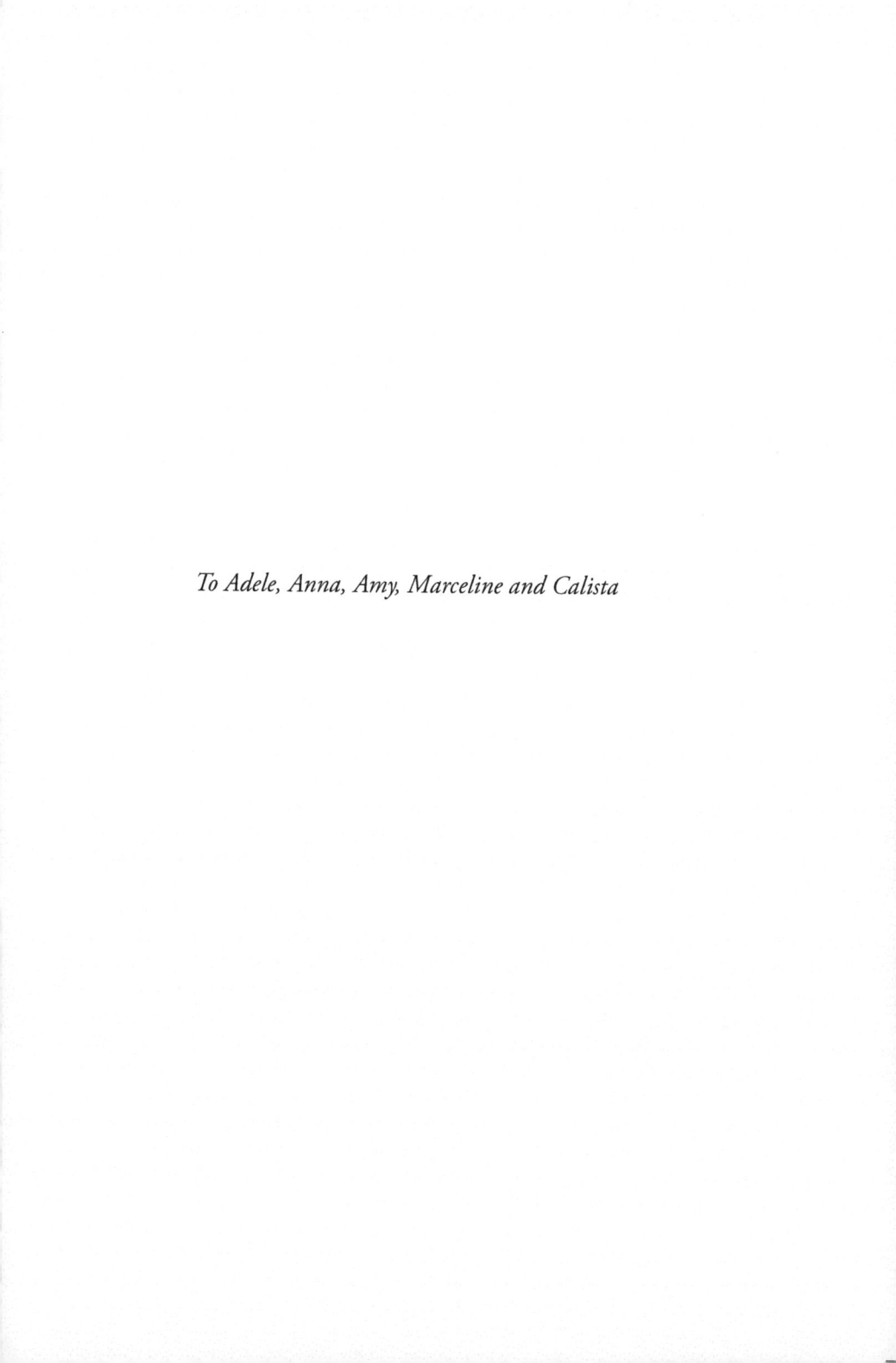

To Adele, Anna, Amy, Marceline and Calista

Preface

Hundreds, if not thousands, of psychotherapy methods have been described. If you have a very liberal mind, you can rejoice in such an "offer": *A chacun son bonheur!*[1] (as they say in the bazars of France). Indeed, such a profusion, undoubtedly a reflection of the complexity and creativity of the human mind, could be welcomed if we had tools to guide clients in choosing a therapy. However, to our knowledge, there is no unified framework where the different types of therapy can be described, their specificities mapped and their indications outlined.

In fact, each school of therapy is rather accustomed to developing on its own account, each claiming to be well founded in clinical experience. The universe of psychotherapies seems to the naive psychology student somewhat compartmentalized between the worlds of these different schools. In particular, a deep canyon seems to separate the bases of cognitive-behavioural therapies from those of psychodynamic or existential therapies. Some build on experimental psychology, others on intuitions about subjective life and the experience of the relationship.

---

[1]"To everyone's happiness".

The person-centred approach may offer a bridge across this canyon, being concerned both with rooting in science and relying on subjective experience. The fundamental attitudes put forward by Rogers—empathy for the subject's inner world, fundamental trust in his/her resources, congruence within the therapist's world—whilst they have inspired all schools of therapy, have so far been unlikely to achieve precise scientific operationalization.

However, advances in cognitive science today make it possible to rely on precise and rigorous tools, supported experimentally, whilst at the same time drawing on the most fertile insights from psychodynamic or existential approaches. For example, it has become possible to propose much more precise constructions of the notion of the *inner world*, as we will show in this book. It is no longer a utopia to envisage a unified framework where the models proposed by the various psychotherapy schools can be integrated, or even develop "tailor-made" therapeutic methods targeted according to the clients' inner worlds. New fields may even have to be explored in psychopathology and psychotherapy, since contemporary cognitive science makes it possible to explore new dimensions of mental life that have hitherto largely escaped scientific knowledge, such as love, imagination, art or scientific creativity itself.

The aim of this book is to propose the first steps towards a *cognitive-psychodynamic* approach. After recalling the current context of psychotherapy in Chapter 1, we will specify what cognitive science can bring today to better ground the understanding of the human mind. In Chapter 2, we will look at the contribution of cognitive science to understanding mental processes and psychological distress. Chapters 3 and 4 will look at human motivation and how our brain represents the past to create an inner world. We will then propose, in Chapter 5, an in-depth approach to the inner worlds, in order to demonstrate the contribution that a cognitive-psychodynamic approach can make to improve support for major types of psychological distress. We will expand on this in Chapters 6–8, applying our proposals to three of the main issues faced by clients, namely depression, trauma and anxiety. In Chapters 9–11, we will outline some of the most exciting perspectives opened by the developments of cognitive science to better understand navigation in mental worlds and better help human beings to face its dangers. Finally, in Chapter 12, we will summarize our key ideas and suggest directions for future developments in inner travel and therapy.

Bristol, UK   Tony Ward
Paris, France   Arnaud Plagnol
May 2019

Acknowledgements

We would like to thank our respective universities, the University of the West of England, Bristol, and Université Paris 8, St. Denis, France, for their support over many years. We would also like to thank our colleagues in psychology and the many students we have worked with, who have helped us to reflect on and refine our ideas. At Paris 8, we would especially like to thank the successive directors of the Laboratoire de Psychopathologie et Neuropsychologie, Michèle Montreuil and Marie-Carmen Castillo, for their support of innovative research over many years. Finally, we would like to thank all the clients we have worked with in many different settings, who have helped us to develop our clinical ideas and theories. We have felt privileged to be able to meet the inner worlds of our clients and in turn to have our own inner worlds changed by the encounter. We are also grateful to the review *Annales Médico-Psychologiques*, Dr. Mirabel-Sarron and Dr. Nicolas Delrue for allowing us to take up in Chapters 7 and 8 some of the cases already mentioned in this journal (note that in the text, previously published case material is identified where relevant— all other case vignettes are an anonymized amalgamation of issues adapted from a number of clients).

Contents

List of Figures

Chapter 6

Chapter 9

List of Tables

1

The Psychotherapeutic Landscape at the Start of the Twenty-First Century

1 The Origins of Psychotherapy

The origins of our modern form of "talking cure" are usually traced back to Sigmund Freud, beginning with his seminal publication on the origin of hysteria. This was co-authored with Joseph Breuer and published in 1895. In this, and his many subsequent publications, Freud laid out his proposals for the method of psychoanalysis. Key notions included the idea that much of human motivation operates at an unconscious level, and that different unconscious forces interact to determine our behaviour. This latter point was captured through the term "psychodynamic". These explanations of human behaviour and motivation put forward by Freud and his many successors remain influential in the field of psychotherapy. This is the profession which developed from Freud's ideas and whose practitioners attempt to ameliorate psychological distress in clients through a process of dialogue.[1]

---

[1]Note that in this book we will use the term "client" to refer to people that access therapy. We will use the term "patient" where this was used by the authors of research studies we reference.

© The Author(s) 2019
T. Ward and A. Plagnol, *Cognitive Psychodynamics as an Integrative Framework in Counselling Psychology and Psychotherapy*,
https://doi.org/10.1007/978-3-030-25823-8_1

It is now a little over 120 years since Freud first began to put forward his ideas. In that time, there have been hundreds of other suggestions advanced around the nature of human distress and how to go about alleviating it. The American psychologist, Carl Ransom Rogers, put forward one early set of rival ideas. Rogers trained as a child psychologist in the 1920s and was initially schooled in Freudian thinking. However, in his early practice at the child guidance clinic in Rochester, New York, he began to question this approach. A particular stimulus appears to have been a visit by Otto Rank around 1936, who shared with Rogers some of his current writing (e.g. on "Will Therapy", first published in English in 1936). Rank was for many years a part of Freud's inner circle, but the two split as it became obvious in the 1920s that many of Rank's ideas were at odds with those of Freud. Rank felt, for example, that classic analysis neglected the emotional life of the client. Rogers seemed to have been heavily influenced by Rank, and published his key work, "Client Centred Therapy" in 1951. In this highly influential book, Rogers argued that the primary aim of the therapist should be to offer a warm, accepting space for the client and to maintain a non-judgemental attitude. According to Rogers, clients needed space to explore their issues, without direction from the therapist. The therapist's task in effect is to provide a safe therapeutic space, in which the client can feel fully accepted and understood.

Another American therapist who was also strongly influenced by Otto Rank was Rollo May. May is associated with the "existential" school of psychotherapy. In acknowledging this influence, May wrote that Rank might be considered the first "existential" therapist (May, 1994). According to this school of therapy, the best way for people to make sense of their own existence is through a consideration of their own experiences. It draws upon phenomenology and existential philosophy, with key themes around death, freedom, responsibility and the meaning of life (van Deurzen & Arnold-Baker, 2005).

At the same time that Rogers was developing his distinctive form of Client-Centred Therapy in the 1930s and 1940s, other psychologists, such as B. F. Skinner, were developing Behaviour Therapy, based upon the principles of classical and operant conditioning. The first published use of the term "Behaviour Therapy" was probably in a report written by Lindsley, Skinner, and Solomon (1953). The approach was quickly picked up and developed by practitioners such as James Wolpe and Hans Eysenck (Clark, Fairburn, & Jones, 1997). Techniques such as relaxation training and systematic desensitization were found to be highly effective in helping people to deal with acquired phobias and anxieties. Alongside these developments, in the 1950s and 1960s, Albert Ellis and Aaron Beck were developing their approaches which focussed on people's thought processes. Ellis's version came to be known as Rational Emotive Behaviour Therapy, whilst Beck's was called "Cognitive Therapy". These differed from the earlier pure behavioural approaches, which tended to focus on behaviour and the environment. By the 1970s, the two strands were being combined under the Cognitive Behaviour Therapy, which now included a focus on the environment, precipitating behaviour, thoughts and beliefs.

Thus, over the last 120 years of psychotherapy development, there have been four main strands of theoretical thinking. These begin with Freud's psychodynamic ideas and then move on to client-centred, existential and cognitive behavioural therapies. It is interesting to reflect that the key personnel in each of the latter three strands were to some extent influenced by Freud's original body of work. Rogers and May, however, came to be influenced by Otto Rank, who had broken away from Freud's circle and espoused a different, more "authentic" and relationally present, view of therapy. Ellis and Beck were both initially trained in Freudian approaches, but became disillusioned and moved away from these, towards approaches rooted in a more immediate, here and now, cognitive phenomenology.

These four main approaches to therapy remain influential to this day. People wishing to train in counselling or psychotherapy could choose to enter a training organization which is guided by one or other of these theories. Counselling psychologists are typically trained in two of the four. This leads to a potentially confusing situation for aspiring trainees, of having to decide which school or schools of therapy they wish to train in. On what basis should such people make their decision? Equally, people in psychological distress who decide they might benefit from psychotherapy might be faced with different practitioners who espouse different approaches. On what basis should they choose a therapist? This situation becomes even more complicated when we consider that there are myriad ways in which people have attempted to bring aspects of these different approaches together into some kind of "integrated" approach, which may or may not have their own label. For example, schema therapy (Young, Klosko, & Weishaar, 2003) could be seen as a combination of cognitive and psychodynamic ingredients (see Chapter 4 for more on this approach).

The aim of this book is to argue the case that cognitive science can be put forward as a strong basis in which to ground a unified, comprehensive account of therapy. To develop this argument, it will be useful to consider in a little more depth the key insights from these four different strands of therapy. This will enable us to consider what is unique to each and where they overlap. From this overview, we will suggest what some of the essential ingredients of effective psychotherapy might be. Having reached this vantage point, we can then go on to consider the extent to which cognitive science can offer a convincing framework for psychotherapy.

2   Key Elements of Psychodynamic Thought—The Importance of Early Experience, Unconscious Phenomena and Defence Processes

A key feature of psychodynamic thinking is the importance placed on the role of our early experience in influencing and shaping our later adult lives. In their early years, human infants experience a massive amount of growth and development. In the first few months, they are totally dependent upon their parents or guardians for all of their needs. They rely on adults to feed, clean and soothe them. At this early stage, when they have not yet mastered the ability to control their muscles and move around, they have limited means in which to influence their environment. However, right from the moment of birth they are able to signal their distress through crying. Research has also shown that infants are able, from a very early stage, to distinguish human faces within their environment. This is illustrated through the observation that they will preferentially direct their gaze towards such stimuli (Bushnell, 2001; Haan, Pascalis, & Johnson, 2002). During the act of feeding, they will look towards their mother's face and seek eye contact. It is believed that these early interactions between mothers and their infants are important in building up the early bond between them (Bowlby, 2008). This is then linked to the infant's development of a later sense of attachment—in other words how secure the infant feels in their relationship with their parents, and the extent to which they can tolerate their parents being absent for short periods. The sense of attachment has been shown to be important in shaping children's early relationships and behaviour. Its influence, however, extends much further than this, into adulthood and our adult relationships (Sroufe, 2005).

Given how important our early years are in setting us up for our future adult lives, it is interesting to note that as adults we have very little recollection of this period. When people are asked to give details of their earliest memories, people often struggle to think of anything much before the age of around four years. For many people, this memory blank for their earliest experiences can extend for much longer, often up to the age of around seven years. Before the age of four, memories tend to be extremely fleeting and brief. This phenomenon whereby people can recall very little detail of the earliest years is referred to as "infantile amnesia" (West & Bauer, 1999). Various theories have been put forward as to why we have such little recall of this early phase of our lives. For example, it has been suggested that as adults much of our memory recall is verbally mediated. In our early years, our language skills are just developing, and thus, the rich linguistic tapestry may not yet exist in which memories can be embedded and thus made available for future recall. As is well known, Freud himself explained childhood amnesia by powerful mechanisms of repression defence, a fundamental notion for psychodynamic thought (see Bauer, 2015; Erdelyi, 2006).

Despite the fact that much of our early experience is inaccessible to future conscious recall, a considerable amount of this experience does remain with us and becomes an integral part of our future lives. We learn complex motor skills such as walking, running and using a pen. We naturally and seemingly without effort acquire the language spoken by those people around us. Clearly, these skills and knowledge are retained in the brain for future use, and this information is encoded in a different format to discrete memories which can be subject to conscious recall (Cowan, 1998). Psychologists have reflected the difference in these types of representation through terms such as "implicit" or "procedural" learning (Baddeley, 2004). The word implicit suggests a type of knowledge or memory process which operates without conscious awareness, whilst procedural refers to our memory for skills or "how to do things". A clear example of procedural memory would be riding a bicycle. Many people are able to do this from an early age, without being able to verbalize quite how they do it.

In addition to learning practical skills and language, our behaviour is also influenced by our environment. We have already mentioned how infants from a very early age are attuned to human faces. Children are also aware of the moods and behavioural styles of the people around them. As will be discussed in the next chapter, we now know that there is a basic brain mechanism which helps us to relate to the mood state of other people. This involves specialist brain cells which have been termed "mirror neurons" (Iacoboni, 2009). Thus, children will learn how their own behaviour may impact upon the moods and emotional states of their carers. They may seek to behave in particular ways which will curry favour with those around them. They may also come to imitate the behaviours and coping styles of the people they observe at close quarters. Children will, therefore, build up complex behavioural repertoires which determine how they will behave and respond to others within their social milieu. Different authors have used a variety of terms to describe these ways of relating. For example, they have been termed "patterns", "templates" or "procedures" (Huprich, 2010; Lemma, 2003). Another term which has been used frequently by many theorists is "object relations". The term "object" refers to people in our environment with whom we interact, and these early interactions have a profound impact on our personal development (Gomez, 1997).

It can be seen then that much of the important early learning we acquire as infants is in the form of procedures, skills and ways of being. Whilst these are things which will have profound impact on our competencies and the kind of person we are, they are not things which we can necessarily verbalize or that we tend to be particularly conscious of on a moment by moment basis. For example, as a child one of our parents may have been a very strict disciplinarian. Over the years, we may have come to recognize that they were more prone to anger when they were in a particular mood or in certain circumstances. At times, therefore, we may have been quite anxious as we recognized that their mood and the circumstances would likely predispose them to an outburst of anger at the smallest infringement. As an adult, we may have completely new relationships with people outside of our families. At times, some of these people might provoke a feeling of anxiety in us. We might not necessarily be aware that this is because this person is recreating some of the same circumstances that provoked our early childhood anxiety. For example, we might be picking up their mood state, or recognize similar circumstances being recreated to those we experienced as a child. The way in which patterns of our early relating as children can play out in our later adult relationships is referred to as "transference" (Lemma, 2003). People are often completely unaware of this process taking place. If they are reflective, they may become aware, over a period of years, as the same pattern is repeated across a number of different relationships and different circumstances.

The preceding discussion leads us on to another set of important concepts. The term "consciousness" is generally taken to refer to our immediate current awareness of our external and internal environment. As will be discussed in the following chapter, the amount of information we can be aware of at any instant in time is extremely limited. Conscious contents are continually shifting as our attention moves from one thing to another. As our attention shifts, the immediate previous contents rapidly fade, but an awareness remains for a brief period of time (Logie, 2011). For example, you are very aware of each word you are reading in this sentence as you move along. At the same time, you retain an impression of the other sentences you have just read in this paragraph. You may be aware of other thoughts or associations you had as you were reading earlier parts of this chapter. If you are a practitioner, you may have remembered a piece of client work that you did in which transference issues were a central part, in response to the previous discussion. If you didn't, maybe reading the previous sentence has brought such a client to mind now. This illustrates a further point. Aspects of our previous experience which are not currently in mind can be accessed and retrieved later (Khader et al., 2007). In traditional psychodynamic terms, information which is not currently conscious can be brought back into our conscious awareness. For example, many practitioners of counselling and psychotherapy are able to recall aspects of the first piece of client work they ever did. However, people who have practised for many years and worked with perhaps hundreds of different clients may struggle to recall much about the detail of those individual cases. Giving a detailed, blow by blow, account of individual sessions is likely to be nigh on impossible. So, although the detail of much of our day-to-day experience may be available to recall for a period of time, over the years it may become lost and inaccessible. At that point, the information has become unconscious. In fact, our ability to recall the day-to-day trivia of our lives is remarkably poor. Even days which at the time may have seemed quite significant will fade with the passage of time. For example, if you think back to five years ago, what can you remember about the details of your birthday? (of course, if it was a significant year you may remember rather more). In addition to this, procedural type memories such as how we are with other people in relationships may be difficult or impossible to verbalize and operate at a level below conscious awareness for much of the time. There is a further complication in that there is not a straightforward split between conscious and unconscious processes. For example, although we may not be able to verbalize quite what is going on in a current relationship, we might have a sense that something is unfolding in a different way. This relationship might not feel the same as others, or it may seem to have somehow changed. Someone we have felt secure with in the past may have suddenly made us feel uneasy, perhaps because of a comment or a tone in their voice.

Finally, most of us wish to maintain a sense of self-worth and enhance our standing in the eyes of others. When things happen which might disturb this, people use a range of strategies to maintain their self-esteem and manage their desires in line with the constraints of the environment. Such strategies are known as "defence mechanisms" (Schaunberg, Willenborg, Sammet, & Ehrenthal, 2007), a fundamental notion that has a long tradition in the psychodynamic approach since Freud. A common strategy is that of repression, in which people actively avoid thinking about a topic which makes them anxious. There is debate about the extent to which such strategies operate at a conscious or unconscious level (as in Freudian psychodynamics). As we will discuss later in Chapter 3, there is scope for both. On the one hand, people may actively stop themselves thinking about something (suppression). On the other, over a period of time, they may have built up a mental or behavioural repertoire which means they avoid circumstances which would cause them to think about that particular topic. They may be deeply unaware of this strategy playing out in practice.

3   The Person-Centred Contribution

Person-centred therapy was developed by Carl Rogers in the 1930s and 1940s. Rogers original training at Teachers College, Columbia University, included exposure to Freudian ideas, but Rogers became disillusioned in that approach. His recollection of how he became disillusioned includes an account of a client who was a male teenager with fire setting tendencies. Rogers described how he carefully explored the client's motivation, and explained this to them, in terms of sexual impulse and excitement, only to find that it had zero impact on the client's behaviour (Rogers, 1951). Gradually, Rogers evolved a technique which involved listening carefully to each client and trying to understand them from within their own inner world and their own narrative. Rather than attempting to impose an outside, expert-driven, point of view, Rogers aimed to enable each client to feel valued and understood. He was strongly influenced in his thinking by Otto Rank, who visited Rogers and his colleagues in 1936 (Kirschenbaum, 1979). Rank had by this time split from Freud's circle, and moved to the USA, where he was involved in training social workers. Rank had come to see the therapeutic relationship as central to achieving positive outcomes, rather than any attempt to uncover the minutiae of an individual's developmental history (Rank, 1936).

Rogers' approach to therapy came to be characterized by the "core conditions". This is a set of principles which therapists should endeavour to work with, to facilitate client growth. Rogers saw these as essential ingredients of his approach, but also suggested that they were probably universal. In other words, other types of therapy were also likely to be successful to the extent to which they operated according to these principles. The three main principles consist of empathy, genuineness and unconditional positive regard. Empathy means listening carefully to the client's narrative and understanding the client's story from their own perspective, in other words from within the client's inner world (or "frame of reference"). Genuineness means being completely up front with the client and not harbouring hidden thoughts and hypotheses. Unconditional positive regard refers to maintaining a positive attitude towards the client and not being critical or judgemental. Rogers argued that if therapists were successful in providing an environment in which these conditions could be enacted and perceived by clients, then this would enable a strong therapeutic bond to be formed. In such an environment, clients would feel safe to explore their innermost feelings and experiences, and reflection on these experiences could then lead to positive change.

As Rogers recognized, the way of working which he proposed was radically different to how other professionals working in the mental health sphere tended to operate at that time. Practitioners who tended to see the role of expert as central to their approach could struggle to live up to Rogers' ideal. For example, as soon as a practitioner starts to explain a client's problems from within a professional framework, in a way that does not accord with the client's own understanding, then empathy is lost. Such an approach might also be seen by clients as negating their own point of view, and thus communicating a negative judgement that the client cannot grasp their own situation. Finally, if the practitioner tries to impose a way forward which the client is not in agreement with, then this may harm the perception of genuineness.

Given that Rogers' approach involves little technique other than providing an environment in which the core conditions can be enacted and perceived, it follows that clients must have within themselves the capacity for positive therapeutic change. Rogers termed this the "actualising potential"—the notion that we all have a tendency to move towards growth and work towards becoming all that we are capable of.

Rogers also developed a theoretical view of how people come to feel a sense of mental disequilibrium, and how therapy works to correct this. Rogers proposed that our early childhood environments involve "conditions of worth". These are expectations placed on us by parents and significant others. If we meet these expectations, then we receive love and esteem from these influential people in our lives. This early environment may also include related feedback about ourselves and our characteristics, and this becomes incorporated into our sense of our personality and who we are. Imagine, for example, the child of parents who are accomplished musicians. This child might sense that they will be more valued if they show musical interest and aptitude. In contrast, they may feel rejected if they fail to do so. Being "unmusical" may then become a part of their self-concept.

Rogers suggested that the sense of self we develop can be highly distorted by these processes, so that as an adult our notion of who we are could be very discrepant from our true, or "organismic", self. To take the above example, someone might see themselves as having no musical talent, when in fact given the right instrument and allowed to follow their own interests they might flourish. Where people have a self-concept, which is grossly at odds with their real selves, they are said to be "incongruent". Rogers felt that such a state of incongruence was a precondition for successful therapy (which implies that personal therapy for trainees is not likely to be productive unless they are in such a state themselves).

The non-directive stance of the person-centred approach is certainly a challenge to most other schools of therapy. The standard critique of the Rogerian position revolves around the extent to which the provision of the core conditions is, by itself, necessary and sufficient. This question appears to have been partly answered from within the person-centred camp itself, towards the end of Rogers' time as an active therapist. In the 1960s, Rogers and colleagues attempted to carry out a trial of person-centred methods for people with severe and enduring mental illness, including schizophrenia. The trial does not appear to have been a success and ended in some acrimony (Kirschenbaum, 2007; Rogers, Gendlin, Kiesler, & Truax, 1967).

4   Cognitive and Behavioural Approaches

Behaviour therapy was developed in the 1950s, based on the theories of learning developed in psychology by Ivan Pavlov and B. F. Skinner (Pinel, 2013). Pavlov developed the theory of classical conditioning, whereby stimuli which provoke a reflex response can come to be associated with other stimuli. Thus, someone bit by a dog could develop an anxiety and fear of all dogs, since the stimuli of a future innocuous dog will provoke the same earlier reaction from the original incident. Skinner's work on operant conditioning showed how behaviour could be shaped and modified through the application of different types of reinforcement. Thus, positive reinforcement will lead to an increase in a particular behaviour. Both classical and operant conditioning have been applied to various states of psychological distress, including anxiety and depression. In relation to anxiety for example, training someone to maintain a relaxed state whilst exposed to a fearful situation has been shown to be an effective way of overcoming fears and phobias, through a process known as extinction in the face of repeated exposure.

Cognitive therapy was developed by Aaron Beck in the 1960s and has many similarities with the approach of Albert Ellis who developed Rational Emotive Behaviour therapy in the 1950s (Beck, 1979; Ellis & Dryden, 2007). Both Ellis and Beck developed their approaches after initially being trained in, and then becoming disillusioned with, psychoanalysis. In his work with depressed clients, Beck noticed that their thinking tended to be characterized by "negative automatic thoughts". These often involved themes of self, world and future. Beck was drawn to the emerging cognitive theories of his day, including Piaget's notion of schemas. He suggested that the negative automatic thoughts seen in clients were a consequence of many years of learning, resulting in schematic memory structures which reflected their core beliefs. People that have developed such negative schemas have a vulnerability which can later be triggered by negative events and stress, leading to negative automatic thoughts and depression.

From the 1970s, the two approaches of behavioural and cognitive therapy were gradually brought together under the term "cognitive behaviour therapy" (Sheldon, 2011).

5   Questions of Existence

A fourth major approach to therapy assumes that much human doubt and anxiety can be traced back to fundamental concerns about what it is to be human and the paradoxes of the human condition. Rooted in the existential philosophies of writers such as Kierkegaard and Nietzsche, key therapists who have developed and promoted this approach include Emmy van Deurzen (Deurzen & Arnold-Baker, 2005) in the UK and Irving Yalom in the USA (Yalom, 1980).

A key issue from the existential perspective is how we derive meaning and purpose in our lives. As human beings, our life span is limited. Whilst some of us may live to be very old, many others of us will not. Given the fleeting nature of our existence, how do we make sense of our lives, and use our time to the best possible advantage? How do we cope with the inevitability of human frailty and weakness? How do we live our lives productively, knowing that ultimately our fate lies in death? (see Irving Yalom [2011], for an extended reflection on this theme).

6   Differences Between Therapies and Schoolism

In the previous sections, we have surveyed the main strands of thought which have developed in psychotherapy in the past 100 years. The initial impetus came from the psychodynamic position, followed by the person centred. From within psychology, the behavioural approach of the 1940s and 1950s was applied to a range of problems. Following the cognitive revolution of the 1950s and 1960s, the cognitive tradition emerged, and in the 1970s this was combined with behaviourism resulting in the cognitive behavioural approach. Alongside these, the existential approach was developed, with its emphasis on the nature and concerns of what it is to be human, and the paradoxes of the human condition (Freedheim et al., 1992).

These various views on therapy clearly have some similarities. For example, they all envisage someone that has chosen to train and gain experience as a therapist sitting alongside and attempting to help people suffering from psychological distress. It could be argued that whilst all approaches see this therapeutic relationship between therapist and client as important, some see it the central concern, especially the person-centred approach. Other schools of thought suggest that the activity of the therapist in the relationship is also important. This could be offering interpretations of current concerns in the light of past experience, in the case of psycho-dynamic, or encouraging the client to explore how they achieve meaning and sense in their lives in the existential. The cognitive behavioural approach is probably the one which promotes the greatest amount of therapist activity, and this can include setting clients tasks and homework to complete outside of sessions, plus carrying out specific interventions in sessions, such as relaxation training.

We can see, therefore, that the approaches differ in the extent to which they place the relationship at the centre of the therapeutic endeavour and the extent to which they encourage the therapist to be active in the relationship.

When we think about the concerns of clients, they are generally mul-tifaceted. Many will have aspects of their narrative which stem from their early experiences. These may include the messages given to them by their caregivers, either overtly or more subtly. It could include early traumatic experiences, which may stem from abuse. As adults, our cli-ents may be plagued by self-doubts, low self-esteem, and continuous negative thoughts about themselves and their lives. They may strug-gle to make sense of their lives and experience a lack of coherence and direction. In exploring such issues, clients will benefit from a safe space, with a therapist that they feel values them and does not judge them in any way. We can see, therefore, how each of the different therapeutic approaches can have something useful to contribute to the work with a typical client. A frequent analogy often used is the Indian folktale about the four blind men and the elephant. When asked to describe what is in front of them, each feels a different part of the elephant, and thus gives a different description of what they can feel. Each feels that they have the true picture and cannot understand why the others seem to have such different impressions (see [Stiles, 2007], for one application of this folktale to psychotherapy). Would it not make sense therefore if thera-pists were open to ideas from the different schools of therapy?

Historically, the problem has been that therapists have often been trained on courses and programmes which specialize in only one of the various approaches. The people training them have tended to be steeped in that approach, which they are committed to. Consequently, if other approaches are referred to, this is often in a negative and critical light. Proponents from within each school believe that they have the truth, and other approaches are at fault (and might even be dangerous!). Thus, psychodynamic practitioners will criticize the cognitive behavioural camp for not paying sufficient attention to people's early experience. In reverse, the cognitive behaviourists will say that psychodynamic practitioners put too much emphasis on unconscious processes, which clients might find disempowering.

In trying to arbitrate between the different therapeutic schools and approaches, there have been various attempts over the years to marshal the available evidence, to see if it supports one form of therapy over another. One early and prescient view on this was published by Rosensweig (1936). Rosensweig suggested that the techniques which therapists put forward for why a particular approach is effective may not in fact be the real reason for efficacy. He predicted that in fact all therapies are likely to be effective to some degree, and that this reflects the extent to which they all share common factors—such as the offering of a facilitative, helping relationship with a fellow human being. This notion which Rosensweig put forward has become known as the Dodo bird hypothesis. In Lewis Carrolls "Alices Adventures in Wonderland", at one point the Dodo bird exclaims "all have won, and all shall have prizes". Since Rosensweig, various authors have reaffirmed the validity of the hypothesis, for example Luborsky (1995) and a more recent follow-up (Luborsky et al., 2002). Wampold and Imel (2015) published one of the most comprehensive and thorough reviews of all the evidence around the effectiveness of psychotherapy, concluding that the evidence shows that all therapies are effective, and that the crucial common ground between them is the offering of a therapeutic relationship (the exception to this, noted by these authors, is in relation to circumscribed conditions characterized by anxiety, where there tends to be an advantage in favour of cognitive behavioural approaches).

It is, therefore, becoming increasingly recognized that the various schools of therapy each have something valid and worthwhile to contribute. There are myriad suggestions about how one might go about trying to integrate these different perspectives into a single unified approach. For those trained along traditional lines in one of the main therapeutic schools, a suggestion is that they might assimilate other approaches. Gold and Stricker (2001) for example describe how, starting from a base in psychodynamic therapeutic practice, they have incorporated wider perspectives from other models. In contrast, Ingram (2011) suggests that practitioners are trained from the outset to develop holistic formulations for their clients, using clinical hypotheses derived from the different theoretical perspectives. Another approach which has become very popular in the UK has been advanced by Cooper and McCleod (2010). This is based on the philosophical premise of pluralism, which is the view that all approaches are equally valid and worthwhile. Cooper and McCleod describe how different therapeutic approaches and methods can be combined within a collaborative framework. This allows different perspectives to be used together for the benefit of clients, in a way in which client consent and choice is maximized.

In our view, it is commendable that there is now an openness to using different therapeutic traditions together for the benefits of clients. However, there is a risk that the different ways of doing this that are being put forward may create further divisions and schools. A way around this would be to try and construct a generic framework, rooted in basic science and theory. Theoretical integration is often put forward as an ideal, as it will lead to principled and defendable ways of combining different elements. At the same time, it is often criticized as being almost impossible to achieve in practice (Safran & Messer, 1997). We believe however that there has been a significant amount of progress around theory within the general psychological sciences, including around cognition, social functioning and neuroscience. There is, in our view, sufficient consensus and understanding emerging, such that a generic foundation can now be proposed for psychotherapy. This theoretical foundation is sufficiently broad to encompass the whole of human experience and unite the field of therapeutic endeavour. What are the key requirements then if a generic framework is to be successful as a basis for thinking about and developing psychotherapy?

7   The Key Requirements of a Theoretical Framework for Psychotherapy

A successful framework for psychotherapy needs to be able to help us understand people, as well as how they come to experience psychological distress and seek therapy. It will also help us to understand the process of therapy and how it works. In doing these things, it will enable therapists to understand why things work as they do, and also allow us to develop and improve therapy further in the future. We would suggest therefore that a successful framework for psychotherapy will need to cover three important domains, as we will now outline below.

7.1   A Comprehensive Account of Human Development, Experience and Phenomenology

We would argue that being a good therapist requires a comprehensive understanding of human beings, what motivates them, and why sometimes they become discouraged. Each of the traditional schools of therapy goes some way towards articulating this understanding. Rogers viewed people as shaped in their childhood through conditions of worth. The cognitive behavioural tradition draws on learning theory and cognitive psychology to suggest how past experience shapes our mood and thought patterns. The psychodynamic view also sees people as shaped by their past, in particular their relationships. It also emphasizes the point that often people are unconscious of the forces that have shaped them and continue to influence their behaviour. The existential approach looks at the processes by which people look for and need meaning in their lives.

There is undoubtedly truth in all of these different traditions and approaches to psychotherapy, and a new comprehensive framework should be able to accommodate them all. It should also be able to explain how these processes change through development and the lifespan and how they give rise to psychological distress.

7.2   An Account of Human Relationships

It could be argued that this aspect is part of the area outlined above; in other words, it could be subsumed under our overall understanding of human beings and how they develop. We think its importance is worth emphasizing as a separate heading. This recognizes that on the one hand, the reason many of our clients come to therapy is because of issues around their relationships with other people. On the other, it recognizes that therapy itself is fundamentally a relational process, involving two human beings interacting together, often over prolonged periods of time. Thus, relationships are often a part of the subject matter of what is discussed in therapy, whilst at the same time a crucial ingredient which may determine the eventual success or otherwise of the enterprise.

The traditional therapeutic approaches have all had something to say about relationship. For Rogers (1951), the therapeutic relationship was the central concern, and he wrote extensively about what effective therapeutic relationships should look like. Similar discussions can be found in each of the other approaches (e.g. Gilbert & Leahy, 2007; Lemma, 2003; Yalom, 1980)

7.3   An Account of the Therapeutic Process

Finally, a successful framework needs to suggest why and how psychotherapy works. This is important to help practitioners think about how what they do is helpful to clients, as well as to guide developments in the future about how therapy can be made more effective.

Again, each of the traditional approaches has had something to say about this, and the answers they provide differ according to their theoretical take on what underlies human distress. For Rogers (1951), the therapeutic relationship was the single key ingredient, whereas in cognitive therapy Beck (1979) felt its important that depressed people should be able to recognize and deal with their negative automatic thoughts. The psychodynamic approach sees value in helping people become aware of past influences on their behaviour, in particular through the phenomena of transference and it's interpretation (Lemma, 2003), whilst existential practitioners work with clients to explore the sense of purpose and meaning in their lives (Yalom, 1980).

Again, our own view is that there is value to all of the suggestions being put forward by these different traditional schools of therapy.

8   Concluding Remarks—The Cognitive Psychodynamic Approach, a Unified Framework for Psychotherapy

In this chapter, we have reviewed the main traditional approaches to psychotherapy. We have seen how they each have come up with explanations of the human condition. They each have a position on human distress and how to work with this in psychotherapy. It can be difficult to arbitrate between these different positions and find a principled way in which they can be combined.

Our suggestion is that psychological science has now reached a point where we have a deep, holistic understanding of the human condition and human distress. We can, therefore, consider to what extent the traditional therapeutic approaches are consistent with this evidence. From such a synthesis, a new comprehensive framework can be put forward. This will lead to increased insights into the therapeutic process and lead to further developments and refinements in the future. To evaluate whether we have been successful in this endeavour, we will again come back to this list of key ingredients. To what extent does such a framework help us to holistically understand human beings? To what extent does it help us to understand the nature of human relationships and the role of relationship in therapy? To what extent does it help us to think about, and further refine, the process of therapy? We will return to these questions at the end of Chapter 5.

We argue that such a framework for psychotherapy is possible. As we will further justify in a later chapter, we are inclined to call this framework a "cognitive psychodynamic approach". This reflects the fact that on the one hand, much of our current understanding of how we are affected by our experience and learning comes through the field of cognitive neuroscience. At the same time, modern psychology recognizes that a significant amount of human information processing takes place at an implicit or unconscious level. We are, therefore, all subject to myriad influences from our past and inclined to play out patterns of behaviour of which we are only dimly aware. This aspect we term "psychodynamic". The combination of understanding how the brain/mind processes and represents information whilst at the same time being subject to unconscious and implicit processes is therefore *cognitive psychodynamic*.

In the next chapter, we will go on to look at the cognitive science which underpins our current knowledge of human phenomenology, in terms of both our thought processes, and the role of emotion. We will then go on, in Chapter 3, to look at the drivers behind human behaviour, i.e. what it is that makes us get up in the morning and keep going. This will be linked to views about human distress. Next, in Chapter 4, we will look at the human representational systems. What of our past experience are we able to recall? How does our past experience shape us and influence our behaviours even without us being aware of it? We will then consider what all of this means for a cognitive psychodynamic view of therapy in Chapter 5.

Points to Ponder

- If you are a therapist or training to be one, which models of therapy have you or are you being trained in?
- Did you choose to train in these specific models? Or was it serendipity?
- Did your training cover a specific model, or several? Or were you trained to work from an integrative perspective right from the start?
- If you have experience of working with clients, do you feel that your way of working enables you to facilitate change for most of them? Are there any particular client issues where you feel you could usefully add other therapeutic strings to your bow?
- If you work with several different models, how have you gone about bringing these together? Have you followed a specific path to combining them?

- What additional training or personal development do you envisage in the future? How will you incorporate this into your existing way of working?
- Some people are happy to combine different ways of working without worrying too much about the principles for doing this, which is often referred to as eclecticism. Others feel that bringing different models together needs to be more principled and opt for one of the different types of integration, such as assimilative or theoretical integration. How do you see yourself in terms of this continuum?

References

Baddeley, A. D. (2004). *Your memory: A user's guide*. New York, NY: Carlton Books.

Bauer, P. J. (2015). A complementary process account of the development of childhood amnesia and a personal past. *Psychological Review, 122*(2), 204–231.

Beck, A. (1979). *Cognitive therapy of depression*. New York: Guilford Press.

Bowlby, J. (2008). *A secure base: Parent-child attachment and healthy human development*. New York: Basic Books.

Bushnell, I. W. R. (2001). Mother's face recognition in newborn infants: Learning and memory. *Infant and Child Development: An International Journal of Research and Practice, 10*(1–2), 67–74.

Clark, D. M., Fairburn, C. G., & Jones, J. V. (1997). *The science and practice of cognitive behaviour therapy*. Oxford: Oxford University Press.

Cooper, M., & McLeod, J. (2010). *Pluralistic counselling and psychotherapy*. London, New York, and Delhi: Sage.

Cowan, N. (Ed.). (1998). *The development of memory in childhood*. London: Psychology Press.

Ellis, A., & Dryden, W. (2007). *The practice of rational emotive behavior therapy*. New York: Springer.

Erdelyi, M. H. (2006). The unified theory of repression. *Behavioral and Brain Sciences, 29*(5), 499–511.

Freedheim, D. K., Freudenberger, H. J., Kessler, J. W., Messer, S. B., Peterson, D. R., Strupp, H. H., & Wachtel, P. L. (1992). *History of psychotherapy: A century of change*. Washington, DC: American Psychological Association.

Freud, S., & Breuer, J. (1895). *The standard edition of the complete psychological works of Sigmund Freud, volume II (1893–1895): Studies on hysteria*. London, UK: The Hogarth Press and the Institute of Psycho-Analysis.

Gilbert, P., & Leahy, R. (2007). *The therapeutic relationship in the cognitive behavioral psychotherapies*. London: Routledge.

Gold, J., & Stricker, G. (2001). A relational psychodynamic perspective on assimilative integration. *Journal of Psychotherapy Integration, 11*(1), 43–58.

Gomez, L. (1997). *An introduction to object relations*. New York: New York University Press.

Haan, M. D., Pascalis, O., & Johnson, M. H. (2002). Specialization of neural mechanisms underlying face recognition in human infants. *Journal of Cognitive Neuroscience, 14*(2), 199–209.

Huprich, S. K. (2010). *Psychodynamic therapy: Conceptual and empirical foundations*. London: Routledge.

Iacoboni, M. (2009). Imitation, empathy, and mirror neurons. *Annual Review of Psychology, 60,* 653–670.

Ingram, B. L. (2011). *Clinical case formulations: Matching the integrative treatment plan to the client*. Hoboken, NJ: Wiley.

Khader, P., Knoth, K., Burke, M., Ranganath, C., Bien, S., & Rösler, F. (2007). Topography and dynamics of associative long-term memory retrieval in humans. *Journal of Cognitive Neuroscience, 19*(3), 493–512.

Kirschenbaum, H. (1979). *On becoming Carl Rogers*. New York: Delacorte Press.

Kirschenbaum, H. (2007). *The life and work of Carl Rogers*. Ross-on-Wye, UK: PCCS Books.

Lemma, A. (2003). *Introduction to the practice of psychoanalytic psychotherapy*. Chichester: Wiley.

Lindsley, O., Skinner, B.F., & Solomon, H.C. (1953). *Studies in behavior therapy* (Status Report I). Walthama, MA.: Metropolitan State Hospital.

Logie, R. H. (2011). The functional organization and capacity limits of working memory. *Current Directions in Psychological Science, 20*(4), 240–245.

Luborsky, L. (1995). Are common factors across different psychotherapies the main explanation for the dodo bird verdict that "everyone has won so all shall have prizes"? *Clinical Psychology: Science and Practice, 2*(1), 106–109.

Luborsky, L., Rosenthal, R., Diguer, L., Andrusyna, T. P., Berman, J. S., Levitt, J. T., ... & Krause, E. D. (2002). The dodo bird verdict is alive and well—Mostly. *Clinical Psychology: Science and Practice, 9*(1), 2–12.

May, R. (1994). *Existence*. Lanham, MD: Jason Aronson.

Pinel, J. P. (2013). *Biopsychology*. London: Pearson Higher Ed.

Rank, O. (1936). *Will therapy: An analysis of the therapeutic process in terms of relationship* (Reprinted 1978). London: Norton.

Rogers, C. R. (1951). *Client centred therapy*. London: Constable.

Rogers, C. R., Gendlin, E. T., Kiesler, D. J., & Truax, C. B. (Eds.). (1967). *The therapeutic relationship and its impact: A study of psychotherapy with schizophrenics*. Madison: University of Wisconsin Press.

Rosenzweig, S. (1936). Some implicit common factors in diverse methods of psychotherapy. *American Journal of Orthopsychiatry, 6*(3), 412–415.

Safran, J. D., & Messer, S. B. (1997). Psychotherapy integration: A postmodern critique. *Clinical Psychology: Science and Practice, 4*(2), 140–152.

Schauenburg, H., Willenborg, V., Sammet, I., & Ehrenthal, J. C. (2007). Self-reported defence mechanisms as an outcome measure in psychotherapy: A study on the German version of the Defence Style Questionnaire DSQ 40. *Psychology and Psychotherapy: Theory, Research and Practice, 80*(3), 355–366.

Sheldon, B. (2011). *Cognitive-behavioural therapy: Research and practice in health and social care*. London: Routledge.

Sroufe, L. A. (2005). Attachment and development: A prospective, longitudinal study from birth to adulthood. *Attachment & Human Development, 7*(4), 349–367.

Stiles, W. B. (2007). Theory-building case studies of counselling and psychotherapy. *Counselling and Psychotherapy Research, 7*(2), 122–127.

van Deurzen, E., & Arnold-Baker, C. (Eds.). (2005). *Existential perspectives on human issues: A handbook for practice*. London: Palgrave Macmillan.

Wampold, B. E., & Imel, Z. E. (2015). *The great psychotherapy debate: The evidence for what makes psychotherapy work*. New York: Routledge.

West, T. A., & Bauer, P. J. (1999). Assumptions of infantile amnesia: Are there differences between early and later memories? *Memory, 7*(3), 257–278.

Yalom, I. D. (1980). *Existential psychotherapy* (Vol. 1). New York: Basic Books.

Yalom, I. D. (2011). *Staring at the sun: Being at peace with your own mortality*. New York: Hachette.

Young, J. E., Klosko, J. S., & Weishaar, M. E. (2003). *Schema therapy: A practitioner's guide*. New York: Guilford Press.

2

Insights from Cognitive Neuroscience

1   Why Is Cognitive Neuroscience Likely to Be Helpful in Progressing Our Thinking About Psychotherapy?

The previous chapter outlined the main schools of thought which have developed in psychotherapy over the past hundred years. It went on briefly to outline some of the key principles from these various approaches. Many practitioners will recognize the wisdom in the different ideas and will incorporate aspects of each into their work. Like the parable of the four blind men and the elephant, many recognize that each tradition only has a grasp of part of the truth.

Where ideas across the different therapeutic approaches do not conflict, combining them in work with clients can be quite straightforward. For example, one can imagine discussing the existential concerns of a client following a trauma, whilst at the same time discussing the nature of the traumatic memory and its tendency to reappear in the form of flashbacks. However, there is often conflict in how the different schools of thought suggest therapists should proceed. For example,

© The Author(s) 2019
T. Ward and A. Plagnol, *Cognitive Psychodynamics as an Integrative Framework in Counselling Psychology and Psychotherapy*,
https://doi.org/10.1007/978-3-030-25823-8_2

the person-centred approach would suggest that therapists refrain from offering advice or interpretations, whereas interpretations might be central to a psychodynamic approach. As an example, imagine a situation where a client describes a conflict at work with a superior. The person-centred practitioner might reflect on this episode, and the feelings it seems to arouse in the client, whereas the psychodynamic practitioner might also reflect on the similarities with the client's previous accounts of their relationships with one of their parents.

In situations where different therapeutic schools of thought seem to be suggesting different ways of proceeding, how are we to make sense of these differences? How can we arbitrate between them and decide on the best approach? Each school of thought will be able to cite clinical case descriptions and, possibly, the results from studies such as clinical trials. However, there are additional lines of evidence which have not traditionally been called on by most therapeutic traditions. One is the extensive weight of findings from experimental studies in cognitive science. Another is the increasing body of work from neuroscience, in terms of how the brain functions. This chapter seeks to outline some of the current findings in these areas and illustrate how they are relevant to psychotherapy. This body of work may help us to further understand and develop the therapeutic process.

2 Overview of the Human Cognitive System

Figure 1 illustrates the main components of the human cognitive system, as described in current cognitive psychology (e.g. see Eysenck & Keane, 2013 for a comprehensive overview of the field).

The top section of the diagram, comprising control and working memory processes, concerns current online processing. The capacity of our immediate conscious awareness is very limited. As you are reading this now, you will only retain in your mind the last few words that you have read. If you wish, you can make a conscious effort to keep some of this information active in your mind. You may choose, for example,

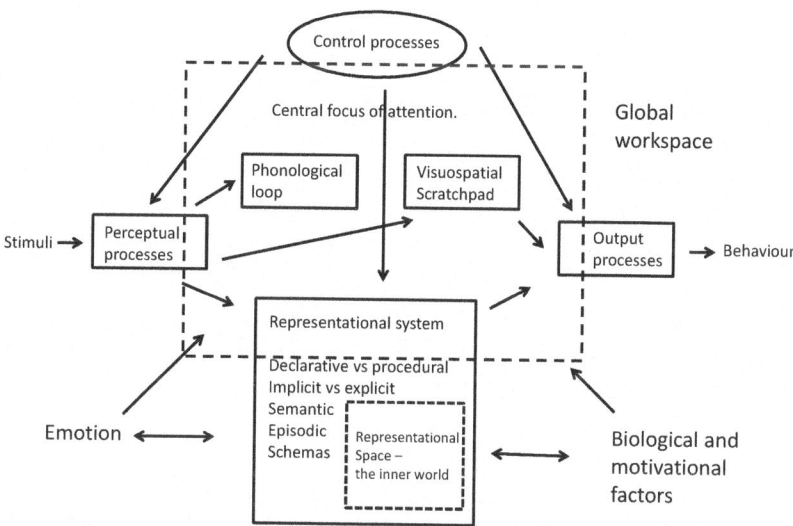

Fig. 1 The human cognitive architecture

to rehearse the words over and over in your minds ear, which Baddeley termed the "phonological loop". Or you may visualize the information using the mind's eye or "visuospatial sketch pad" (Baddeley, 1992). It is tempting to equate this moment to moment awareness with "consciousness". The precise words in the previous paragraph may no longer be available, though you may recall the gist of the meaning. This recall, however, is coming from your long-term, rather than immediate memory. The extent to which information is retained in long-term memory and can be recalled is dependent on a number of factors, including the depth of processing (Craik & Tulving, 1975). We will all have had the experience of reading a book at a point when we are tired and not able to concentrate. After reading a few pages, we may realize they have made no impression on our long-term memory, and we have to go back and read that section again.

The lower part of Fig. 1 consists of representational processes, which deal with how past behaviour, experience and learning are stored in the brain. At a given point in time, much of our past experience will be unconscious, that is to say not actively in mind. Some of that experience may be retrievable, but in fact much of it will not. Past experience that can no longer be recalled can therefore be said to be truly unconscious.

Other processes operate outside of these systems. Our brains enable us to feel and perceive a variety of emotions, and these sensations impact upon the cognitive and control systems. Likewise, there are various biological drives, e.g. around hunger, thirst and sex, which will impact upon our cognition (Pinel, 2013). Linked to these is the motivational system which drives our behaviour and this topic will be more fully discussed in the next chapter. These various influences operate across the different levels of the cognitive system. So, for example, our current motives may not be uppermost in our minds, but they are represented as part of the representational system. To illustrate this point, think for a moment what it is like to engage on a very consuming task such as reading a book. Whilst lost in the narrative, my motives around maintaining strong and loving relationships may not be uppermost at that point (unless of course I am reading a book about how to develop better relationships!). Also, my motives may not always be crystal clear to me. If I have been hurt by someone in a relationship in the past, I may feel for the moment it is better to be by myself. However, the need for companionship could still be an active motive, causing a conflict. One thing which has become clearer from artificial intelligence models in cognitive science is that stored knowledge in the representational system is not inert and passive (Anderson, 1995). Current online processing is influenced at all times by the representational system, in the massively interconnected anatomical structure that is the human brain.

Hence, having suggested that the uppermost part of the diagram in Fig. 1 represents our current, active, processing, which is similar to the notion of consciousness, we can also see that these online processes will be constantly influenced by other systems, including emotion, drives and our goals and motivations. The human cognitive system is therefore intensely dynamic, with our behaviour at any moment being determined by myriad interconnected and interacting systems.

We will now look at some of these systems and influences in more detail.

3 Controlling, Planning and Problem Solving—The Rational, Intellectual, Part of the Mind

The ability to exercise free will and deal with new and complex scenarios could be seen as a hallmark feature of human experience. Being able to control and direct our mental processes is fundamental to how we go about this. We can illustrate this through reference to the cognitive architecture illustrated in Fig. 1. The diagram shows on the left-hand side stimuli from the external world being presented to our cognitive system. These stimuli may consist of visual images, sounds, smells or touch. Our everyday experience is likely to be a complex melange of all these senses. For example, as you are reading this text you will be aware of the pattern of black and white characters on the white printed page. You may also be aware of other stimuli in your surrounding environment. Pause for a moment and reflect on what is going on in your immediate environment. If you are reading quietly in your lounge you might be vaguely aware of the noise of a clock ticking in the background. If you listen carefully, you might be able to hear the sound of birds outside of your window. As you move your attention around, you may become aware of the pressure of your seat pressing on your back. You might have a sensation related to temperature, perhaps feeling neither too hot nor too cold. If you were gardening recently, there might be a faint aroma of cut grass in the air.

At any given moment, you have a choice to make about which of all these available stimuli you will choose to attend to. As you were reading the previous paragraph, you may have looked up from your reading to see what stimuli in your environment you can currently become aware of, prompted by the suggestions given in the text. Some of those suggestions may have prompted other ideas to come to your mind. For example, the suggestion of a freshly mowed lawn may have brought into your mind an image of your garden, or perhaps a favourite park that you used to play in as a child. If you did retrieve such images, then these are clearly not coming from your current environment but from your long-term memory. If you choose to, you can explore these memories in some depth. For example, try closing your eyes and imagine yourself in a favourite garden or park that you knew as a child.

The point being made here is that at any given moment in time we can "choose" what we pay attention to, even if an infinite variety of factors are in play. Such a choice can be voluntary or driven by more unconscious factors (such as in mind-wandering). Moreover, the object of our concentration could be in the external world, but it could equally be an image or sensation we have retrieved from our memories. It could be part of our inner world.

Baddeley and Hitch (1974) put forward a detailed theory of how the cognitive system maintains information in mind over short periods of time, which they referred to as "working memory". As mentioned in the introductory section, information is either retained in a visual format by the "visuospatial sketchpad", or in an auditory format by the "phonological loop". Many everyday tasks could be equally well accomplished using either of these formats. For example, psychologists often test short-term memory by asking people to recite a sequence of digits. Many people given a set of numbers to remember, such as one, three, eight, nine, six, would remember them by repeating them to themselves over and over in their mind. They are thus using the phonological loop, made possible by the existence of a high degree of linguistic competence in most adults. Others however might choose to see the numbers as if on an internal screen, using the mind's eye or "visuospatial sketch pad". Thus, even on a relatively simple task we have choices to make in terms of how we use our working memory. Baddeley and Hitch recognized that they needed to include some kind of decision-making process in their account and they called this the "central executive".

Shallice (1982) was interested in the issue of control processes from a slightly different angle. His focus was on how people go about solving complex novel problems. He hypothesized a mechanism called the "supervisory attentional system". According to Shallice, much of our everyday behaviour is based on very well learnt routines. When we are confronted by a chair for example, we can perform the act of sitting without too much thought. This behaviour is said to be automated and controlled by schemas of our past learning (a schema is an organized body of information retained in memory). When we are confronted by novelty, such as an unusual design of chair which we have not seen before, then we may have to engage in a degree of problem-solving in order to work out what it is we need to do. Such processing is said to be "controlled" and requires a high degree of attention and concentration. Automatic processes on the other hand can proceed virtually without awareness (consider, for example, how a skilled motorist can perform the complex task of driving whilst simultaneously holding a conversation and following directions from a satellite navigation system). This link with solving novel complex tasks suggests that these control processes in the brain may have something to do with intelligence. A number of recent studies have in fact shown that the ability to deal with novel tasks is associated with performance on traditional intelligence tests (Duncan, Burgess, & Emslie, 1995; Roca et al., 2009).

A review by Collette and Van der Linden (2002) summarized a wide array of studies showing that control processes are associated with the

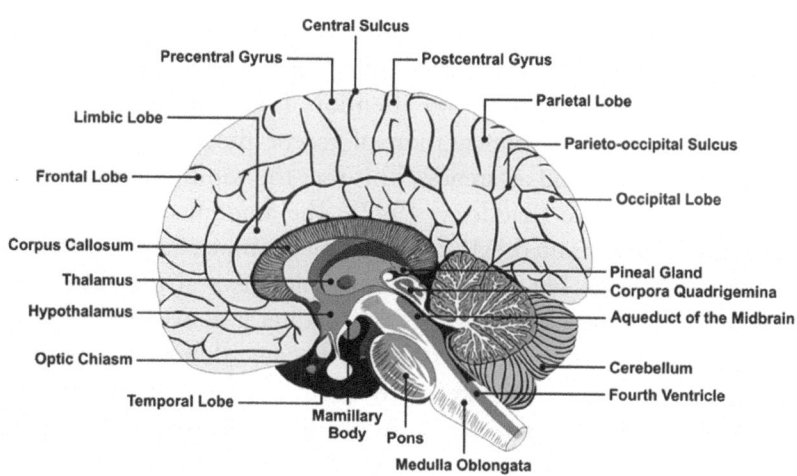

Fig. 2   Cross section of the human brain

prefrontal and parietal parts of the brain, and that these brain regions are involved in the performance of a wide variety of complex tasks (see Fig. 2 for illustration of the main regions of the brain). Other studies supporting this neural basis of working memory and control processes include D'esposito et al. (1995) and Eriksson, Vogel, Lansner, Bergström, and Nyberg (2015). In the latter study, different areas of cortex were identified as being linked to different types of stimuli within immediate awareness. Visual stimuli were associated with the temporal lobe, spatial with the parietal lobe and verbal with both the lateral temporal and the tempo/parietal lobe. Maintenance of material in mind and goal monitoring were associated with the prefrontal cortex.

4   The Limited Capacity of Attention and Immediate Memory

As described above, the human cognitive system is able to orient itself to the external environment through the five main senses of sight, sound, touch, smell and taste. Through control processes located in the frontal part of the brain, we can choose to pay attention to particular stimuli, or change the focus of our attention. If we wish to, we can also choose to maintain a representation of recent processing within our immediate attention and awareness. This uses the working memory processes described above (Baddeley, 1992). The amount of attention we have to pay is very limited. Most people, for example, can easily follow a single conversation but will struggle to follow two at the same time. Whilst driving, most drivers will cease holding a conversation with a passenger if the road conditions suddenly become difficult or complex. Likewise, the amount we can keep actively in mind is very limited. The number of chunks of information we can maintain has been accepted for many years as around about 7 (with a range of 7 ± 2 across the population—Baddeley, 2001).

This section illustrates that the centre of our attention and awareness is very limited and that the contents of this central awareness can come from current direct sensory experience, or from memory. This leads us onto the next main feature of the cognitive architecture, the long-term representation system.

5   The Presenting Past—Long-Term Representation

So far, we have discussed how as humans we experience a constant stream of consciousness, allowing us to be aware of our immediate environment. We are able to reflect on how to achieve our goals and to maintain information at the forefront of our mind using working memory processes.

However, we are not limited to thinking about things in our immediate experience. We can recall events from our past and rely on extensive amounts of past learning in our day-to-day interactions. For example, in reading this sentence, you are deciphering a pattern of black alphabet characters on a white page, which allows you to connect with words and concepts you learned as a child. This acquired knowledge is referred to as semantics. It includes our knowledge of language, both written and spoken, our knowledge of objects and their properties, as well as facts about the world. For example, most UK readers will know why 1066 is an important number but may be less aware of why 1789 is significant in France.

Besides this large amount of semantic learning, we can also recall events from our personal history. Our memory of the day-to-day events is called "episodic memory", whilst autobiographical memory consists of episodes along with knowledge of ourselves, our life stages and future goals (Conway, 1990). Only a fraction of what actually happens to us from day to day is retained in a distinctive form which is accessible to conscious recall. For example, if you choose a random date and year, such as the 11th of February 2011, most people will be able to recall little if anything that might have happened to them at that time (unless of course it just happens to be a significant date for you, such as your birthday, or a date on which something significant and personal happened to you or someone you love).

Whilst recall of routine, everyday, information can be poor, other aspects of our past can be subject to detailed recollection. For example, if we wish to, we can use our minds eye (Baddeley's visuospatial sketch pad) to bring forward an image of our early childhood home. Whilst keeping this image in our minds eye, we may be able to survey the scene. Imagine, for example, a lounge area, perhaps with a table and chair, cupboards, shelves with books, ornaments on a fireplace and so on. Whilst looking at this complex scene retrieved from memory, we will struggle to simultaneously hold another complex image in mind. As soon as we stop trying to hold the image, it will fade back into our memory, to be replaced by whatever we are currently looking at, or some other image drawn from memory.

Details from memory which can be recalled are referred to as explicit memories. Much of our learning remains implicit as already mentioned in Chapter 1. For example, we may have an aversion to a particular food, perhaps acquired in childhood, which affects our behaviour around food choice. However, the original events that led to that aversion may no longer be open to recall.

Memories are typically organized into complex structures, with related information being strongly linked together, such that remembering one thing will lead to associated concepts being activated. If we think of a term such as *cat*, a number of related concepts might spring to mind (such as *dog*, for many people). These memory structures can include a rich tapestry of information, from all our senses, as well as our emotions. Thinking of the term *cat* may well be experienced as positive for cat lovers, or it could evoke sadness where people think of a specific pet they have loved and lost. These complex structures of related material in memory have come to be known as "schemas" (Rumelhart, 2017).

Thus, we can see that the brain retains huge amounts of our past experience and learning, and that across our lives complex memory structures evolve and have an important role in shaping our current and future behaviour. We term this complex set of representation processes and represented contents the "inner world". So important is this to understanding ourselves and our adaption to the outer world that we will devote the whole of Chapter 4 to this topic.

6   The Cognitive Architecture and the Nature of Consciousness

As we have seen, the cognitive architecture suggests that we have an ongoing awareness, whilst we are awake, of external stimuli, currently active memories, immediate goals and our current behaviour. Baars (1994) suggested that our awareness constitutes an inner *mental workspace*, allowing us to bring together our perception of the world, our goals and any relevant memories, e.g. past recollections of how we have previously solved particular problems. Consciousness then, according to Baars, is a mental process which allows us to assemble our mental resources, in order to reflect on our current situation, and direct our behaviour to help us fulfil our wishes in the future. Dehaene and Naccache (2001) put forward very similar ideas around how conscious experience functions as a global workspace. From a phenomenological point of view, what is important is that such a workspace defines the *window of presence* of the inner world, whose content is very limited, as made clear in the above section. A simple analogy would be the way in which an Internet browser window opens on a very limited content of the World Wide Web. Moreover, as the very term "workspace" alludes, much of this content is presented in a visuospatial mode in the visuospatial sketch pad (Baddeley, 1986, 1992) or *spatial field* (e.g. Lyon, Gunzelmann, & Gluck, 2008), or *spatial array* (e.g. Ragni & Knauff, 2013), or *work plan* (Plagnol, 2002, 2004, in press).[1] We will come back in more detail in later chapters to these concepts, which are essential to understanding the construction of an inner world.

However, below this level of awareness, there is a vast array of implicit, schematic processes. These patterns of processing and responding have been conditioned by our past. They may be triggered without us being aware and lead to behavioural responses which unfold automatically, a process termed by Shallice (1982) as "contention

---

[1]*Spatial array* or *spatial field* emphasizes that what is important is the spatial display at a given time, not the usual sensory modality underlying this display. (Blind people have a spatial array in their working memory.) *Work plan* emphasizes that the displayed content is subject to mental processing.

scheduling". The operation of these processes could be seen as "unconscious".

Thus, at a global level, the cognitive architecture of the mind could be seen as compatible with psychodynamic frameworks such as that proposed by Gold and Stricker (2001). These authors suggested that the concerns of their clients could be explained at three levels, which they label as overt behaviour, conscious cognition and unconscious processes. These correspond to the various parts of the cognitive architecture outlined in this chapter. The advantage of the cognitive architectural point of view is that it adds considerable detail, thus allowing client issues to be conceived of in much more depth, which in turn may lend itself to increased therapeutic insight. It may also increase research productivity in terms of generating new hypotheses, which may help drive future developments in therapeutic process. This will be illustrated further in the next chapter, which will consider how traditional Freudian defence mechanisms can be conceived of within the proposed cognitive architecture, and how this may lead to novel therapeutic approaches.

7   The Role of Emotion in Cognitive Processing

In a thorough review, Lazarus (1991) described the range of work in psychology in relation to emotion. In the article, it is suggested that emotion is a product of the interaction between people and their environment, and that these emotional states can be positive or negative. Much of the research produced by Lazarus and colleagues over many years has looked at the issue of how people cope with these negative emotions.

Whilst there are many thousands of words in the English language to denote emotional states, Ekman argued that there are a small number of basic emotions which can be universally recognized. These are reflected in facial expressions (Ekman, 1992). These basic emotional states are *happy, sad, angry, fearful, disgusted* and *surprised*. Cues such as facial expression and tone of voice let us identify emotional states in other people, and it has been suggested that this process occurs at two levels, the cognitive and the empathic (Shamay-Tsoory, Aharon-Peretz, & Perry, 2009). At a cognitive level, we know that certain events will lead people to feel in a particular way, and we can then infer what their emotional state might be. For example, if someone tells us that someone very close to them has just died, we are likely to infer that they will be feeling sad. Similarly, someone in tears is likely to produce the same inference of sadness (though this can be a confusing signal as sometimes people cry tears of joy). However, even without knowing any of the reasons behind how someone else might be feeling, if we see them displaying strong emotion we are likely to sense what this is through a process of empathic resonance. We now know that there are neurons associated with the motor cortex which respond to physical cues in others, leading to the replication of internal states in the perceiver (Schulte-Rüther, Markowitsch, Fink, & Piefke, 2007). Thus, seeing someone in floods of tears is likely to provoke a sensation of sadness in ourselves leading us to identify and even vividly experience the same emotional state of the other person. Given their role in reflecting the actions and emotional states of others, these cells have been labelled as "mirror neurons".

We are thus constantly exposed to reactions and changes in our emotional states, provoked by the environment, and capable of picking up and recognizing these states in the people around us. There seems to be a common set of basic emotions that most people would recognize and label in the same way.

Bagozzi and Pieters (1998) outlines how, when we think about possible future courses of action, we anticipate the likely future emotion this will evoke. This mechanism plays an important role in decision-making processes. Similarly, in a number of articles, Bechara and colleagues have outlined (Bechara, 2004; Naqvi, Shiv, & Bechara, 2006) how bodily states, or somatic markers, can be invoked and play a role in guiding our actions. They suggest that ventromedial prefrontal pathways are important in the brain in making this link between emotions and events. These somatic markers can lead to overt sensations of alarm or pleasure, or covert behaviour, for example a bias to focus on negative aspects of the environment. People with lesions in the ventromedial area appear to have problems in learning from negative events, for example as shown in gambling tasks. These typically allow the person doing the task to experience a good run followed by a sequence of negative trials. Most people tend to stop after a few bad turns. Further evidence shows that control participants will show a galvanic skin response when engaged in risk-taking, but again this is not present in the case of people with ventromedial lesions. In this latter group, emotional information does not seem to be part of the decision-making picture at all. Thus, ventromedial lesions seem to interfere with people's ability to re-experience the emotion of a situation. This is further evidenced by the lack of a physiological response when people are asked to remember happy or sad events, and the same results are found in response to external images.

An example of how this emotional component of decision-making is present in our everyday lives comes from Turner et al. (2003). They describe how school pupil's choices and motivations around what to study and which activities they prefer are influenced by the emotion they experience in relation to each. Pupils that experience maths as anxiety provoking will avoid numerate activities, whilst at the same time they may be drawn to another abstract numerate subject such as physics which they find stimulating and interesting.

Our lives are therefore accompanied by an emotional tone, in response to events happening in our environment. When we think about a possible course of action, this will evoke an anticipated sensation, and this will then have an influence on our decision-making. The outcome of all this is that we will be drawn to actions and activities associated with positive emotions, but we will be reluctant to engage in activities associated with negative emotions. As we will see in the next chapter, which will discuss the topic of human motivation, this overall tendency to either approach situations or avoid them is thought to be a basic principle. It is likely to be an important aspect of the life narratives which clients bring to us in therapy.

8   Fear and the Amygdala

As we noted in the previous section, fear is one of the universal basic emotions that people experience. Fear reactions are triggered very quickly, often with little if any conscious awareness.

This is not surprising, given that these reactions are often aroused by fear-provoking and potentially dangerous stimuli, and our quick reaction could be a matter of life or death.

Consider, for example, someone out walking along a heath, who suddenly happens across something which has the appearance of a large snake. Certain stimuli seem to be hard-wired to provoke fear in humans, perhaps as a result of the proven survival value across the millennia of human evolution. The initial visual stimuli of the snake will be transmitted to the thalamus, from where a signal will be immediately relayed on to the amygdala, ahead of it arriving at the sensory cortex (Pinel, 2013). This will produce a rapid threat response, for example an immediate reaction to freeze. This fast response, involving adrenaline release and preparation for fight or flight happens instantly, even before our conscious awareness has fully caught up with what is happening (see Fig. 3 for illustration of the major structures in the limbic system).

The threat stimulus then reaches the sensory cortex, which also brings in signals from the hippocampus, allowing contextual memories to be activated. Consciously, we become aware that on this heath it is highly unlikely that we would come across a large snake, and in fact, the more we look at it, the snake appears to be an old and twisted branch.

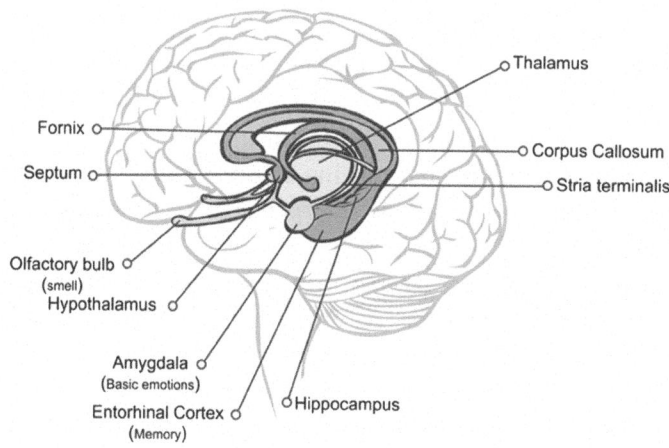

Fig. 3   The limbic system

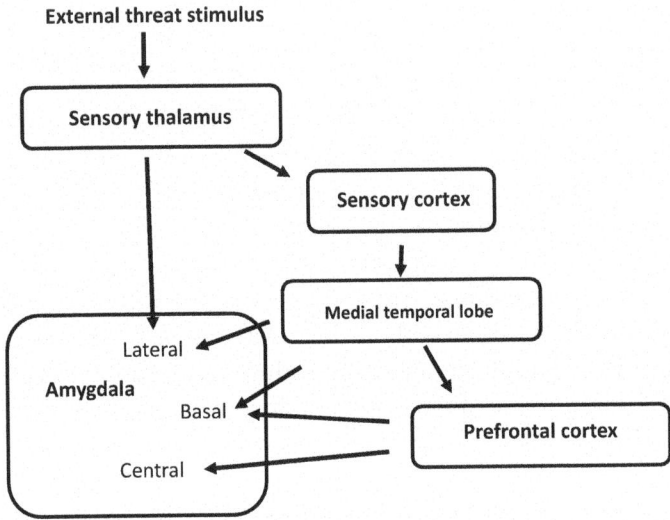

Fig. 4 Information flow to the amygdala

Inhibitory signals are now sent to the amygdala which becomes deactivated, whilst the prefrontal lobes are involved in evaluating the situation and deciding that no further action is needed. This sequence is illustrated in Fig. 4.

We noted above that humans are able to recognize emotions in others, and following on from this, one type of stimuli, which the amygdala is conditioned to respond very strongly to, is fearful, irritated and angry faces (Adolphs, 2008). Linked to this, people with damage to the amygdala may have trouble recognizing emotions in others, with all the attendant consequences for their interpersonal relationships (Adolphs et al., 1999).

The amygdala, therefore, reacts to fear-provoking stimuli, leading to a range of physiological and behavioural responses. However, it can also respond to other stimuli, which have become associated with a fear-provoking stimulus through a process of conditioning. This phenomenon has been thoroughly researched over many years by LeDoux and colleagues (e.g. see Nader, Schafe, & LeDoux, 2000). As mentioned above, the hippocampus will bring information about context and spatial layout to the fearful situation, and these aspects may become conditioned into the fear response. Thus, the fear evoked during a bad car accident could become associated with many aspects of the situation, such as motorways, being a passenger, the noise of passing vehicles and so on. Studies have confirmed the role of the amygdala in conditioned fear responses (Costafreda, Brammer, David, & Fu, 2008) and have also shown that the conditioned stimuli need not actually be conscious (Bryant et al., 2008).

The amygdala is densely connected to other parts of the brain, and thus fear reactions trigger many other responses in other systems. For example, the locus coeruleus is stimulated to release noradrenaline, leading to increased heart rate, whilst the hypothalamus will stimulate the release of corticosteroids and the activating sympathetic nervous system. These somatic markers will then be picked up by the orbitofrontal cortex, as we described above in the section on emotion, and this part of the brain will then ascribe affective meaning to events. These various systems feedback to the amygdala, leading to a positive feedback loop, whereby the brain can become more and more aroused very quickly.

Conditioned fear responses can be stubborn and remain in place for long periods of time, often requiring therapeutic intervention. For example, imagine if someone was involved in a serious road accident, and they now have trouble travelling in cars. If they could bring themselves to be repeatedly exposed to the feared situation, then eventually the fear would subside, a process known as *extinction*. Research suggests that in fact what is happening here is that the orbitofrontal cortex inhibits the fear response, rather than allowing it to build—the original fear memory itself remains intact (Paré, Quirk, & Ledoux, 2004). For example, in people with arachnophobia who have been successfully treated for the condition, physiological responses to the fearful images remain intact even after the fear reaction itself has been controlled (Dilger et al., 2003). Rodrigues, Schafe, and LeDoux (2004) also make the point that stress hormones appear to be able to exacerbate fear reactions. Thus, latent fear can re-emerge under duress, or previously mild and well-controlled fears suddenly become unmanageable.

9   The Role of the Hippocampus

The hippocampus is a horseshoe-shaped structure which runs between the cortices and the brain stem (see Fig. 3). It is important in the formation of new memories and spatial orientation (Hampson, Simeral, & Deadwyler, 1999). Periods of prolonged stress expose the hippocampus to corticosteroids (Sapolsky, Uno, Rebert, & Finch, 1990), and this can lead to degeneration and cell death, leading to increased future vulnerability (Kim & Diamond, 2002). A variety of conditions including post-traumatic stress disorder and depression have been associated with cell loss in the hippocampus (De Lanerolle, Kim, Robbins, & Spencer, 1989). Lower hippocampus volume appears to be linked to deficits in processing short-term memories, in making links to long-term memories, and to vulnerability to psychological trauma (Gilbertson et al., 2002).

The amygdala, therefore, seems to function by rapidly raising attention to possible threats and fear-related stimuli, whilst the hippocampus is about contextualizing this information and letting us process the specifics. Whilst the traumatized car accident victim mentioned above might fear travelling by car, they can access the specifics of the current situation. They can recall that this is not the car they had an accident in, that the conditions are different, and that the nature of the accident they experienced means it is unlikely to happen in quite the same way again.

10   Obsessive-Compulsive Behaviour— A Distinct Type of Anxiety-Related Condition?

The experience of anxiety in the face of repeated compulsion to repeat a particular behaviour, e.g. handwashing, might suggest similarities with the amygdala-based fear circuit we have described above. Research, however, suggests that obsessive-compulsive tendencies have a distinctive basis in the brain. Multiple authors suggest that a neural circuit involving the orbitofrontal cortex, basal ganglia and thalamus is hyperactive (Baxter et al., 1996; Huey et al., 2008). This hyperactivity in this circuit which is involved with behaviour initiation leads to behavioural routines being triggered excessively, and the triggered routines often revolve around themes of aggression, sexuality and hygiene (Saxena, Brody, Schwartz, & Baxter, 1998). Activation in the orbitofrontal cortex is correlated with that in the caudate nucleus for people with obsessive-compulsive behaviour who respond to treatment, with the link being removed following treatment (Saxena et al., 2009). The link was not evident in people with obsessive-compulsive behaviour who did not respond to treatment, which suggests there may be different subtypes of this issue in clients.

11   The Neurobiology of Depression

Finally, in this chapter, we will briefly consider the neurobiological research that has been conducted around depression.

We saw earlier that the frontal lobes of the brain are associated with mental control, planning and problem-solving. It has also been suggested that stronger activation of the left prefrontal cortex (PFC) is associated with increased positive emotion, whereas greater right PFC activation is associated with increased negative emotion. As we shall discuss in the next chapter, left PFC is also associated with approach tendencies and reward, and right PFC with avoidance and punishment (Davidson, 2000). In people with depression, the left PFC is under activated compared to the right PFC (e.g. Debener et al., 2000) suggesting that depressed people may be less inclined to approach positive experiences. Bruder et al. (2001) found that greater asymmetry in favour of activation of the right PFC was associated with poor treatment outcomes with selective serotonin re-uptake inhibitor-type anti-depressants (SSRIs) and thus may be linked to the experience of more negative moods. This asymmetry also extended to more posterior brain regions, suggesting that in these cases there may have been concomitant anxiety. This suggests that anxiety alongside depression may therefore be a predictor of complications with this treatment.

Notwithstanding the noted asymmetries above, the overall level of activation of frontal brain regions tends to be lower in depression. Some studies have linked this to lower volumes of frontal grey matter (Coffey et al., 1993). Hasler, Drevets, Manji, and Charney (2004) noted the substantial volume reductions in people with depression that also had depressed relatives, suggesting a possible genetic link in some instances. From this research, it remains unclear whether reductions in PFC volume are a consequence of prolonged depression, or the initial cause.

The anterior cingulate cortex (ACC) has strong connections to the limbic system, as well as the prefrontal cortex and the motor strip. It tends to be activated by novel situations requiring some kind of choice to be made, where things are not perceived to be progressing according to the desired plan (MacDonald, Cohen, Stenger, & Carter, 2000). As a result, attention is increased and executive functions become more available.

In people with depression, the ACC is chronically under activated (Beauregard et al., 1998; Drevets, Savits, & Trimble, 2008). As a consequence, their response is sluggish, even in the face of situations not progressing satisfactorily or to plan. In effect, people with depression seem to be resigned and they have given up actively trying to intervene in their environment, a situation reminiscent of the learned helplessness phenomenon (see Chapter 6 on depression for more on this). When depression reduces, ACC activation increases (Mayberg et al., 1999) and this is also evident amongst people that respond to pharmaceutical treatment (Mayberg et al., 1997). It has been suggested that the ACC may play an important role in the development of depression, as well as the later expression of symptoms (Drevets et al., 2008).

Thus, both the PFC and ACC play an important role in depression, and it has been suggested (Davidson, Pizzagalli, Nitschke, & Putnam, 2002) that there may be subtypes depending on which area is most implicated, with the PFC subtype being aware of the environmental demands on them not being met but being unable to change their behaviour to meet them, and the ACC type being resigned and not aware of the discrepancy between the environment and their current behaviour. Evidence suggests that the PFC subtype would have the better prognosis (Mayberg et al., 1997). Having said this, it is still very unclear how these brain regions interact, and it could be that the relative activation of different areas changes as the condition progresses.

The hippocampus is known to be reduced in volume in people that are depressed, with studies estimating the reduction between 8 and 19% (Davidson et al., 2002). The amount of reduction seems to correlate with the total length of depressed episodes, rather than age (Sheline, Sanghavi, Mintun, & Gado, 1999). As discussed in the previous section, hippocampus volume is also known to be reduced in other conditions such as post-traumatic stress syndrome, and this might reflect a common role of stress and prolonged exposure to cortisol (Sheline, 2000).

In contrast, new neurons can be formed in the hippocampus, thanks to environmental enrichment (Gould, Tanapat, Rydel, & Hastings, 2000) or anti-depressent intervention (Malberg, Eisch, Nestler, & Duman, 2000).

These findings do not preclude the possibility that people susceptible to depression or post-traumatic stress syndrome start off with smaller hippocampuses, which are then less able to down-regulate and reduce cortisol levels in the face of stress. This is consistent with a study by Gilbertson et al. (2002), who found that hippocampus volume was reduced in both twins where only one had developed post-traumatic stress in response to an environmental incident.

Overall, evidence, therefore, suggests that however it comes about, hippocampus function is impacted in depression, but that this situation can improve with treatment.

Finally, the amygdala has been found to be enlarged in people with depression, probably due to the increased ongoing activation of negative emotional states (Drevets, 2000, 2001). Degree of activation has been correlated to severity of depression, with activation returning to normal following treatment (Abercrombie et al., 1998). The increased activation remains however in those with a family history (Drevets et al., 1992). The amygdala appears to play an important role in the development of depression, especially where it co-occurs with anxiety. The anxiety is thought to develop first, followed by the depression (Nutt, Ballenger, Sheehan, & Wittchen, 2002).

12   Concluding Remarks—What Are the Implications for Psychotherapy?

What are the implications of the neurobiological findings for psychotherapy?

We have seen how the brain responds to threat through a quick and unconscious mechanism that has evolved, linking the thalamus directly to the amygdala. This then provokes an overall anxiety response, which can become generalized and associated with wider aspects of the triggering environment.

Another consistent finding is the impact of severe and chronic stress, which seems to leave people in a vulnerable position due to changes in important structures such as the hippocampus. Heim and Nemeroff (2001) reviewed evidence that people with significant childhood history of trauma responded to a significantly greater extent in response to a stress test as an adult, and that this was further magnified by the presence of current depression.

People experiencing depression may over time cease trying to seek out positive experiences and become more receptive to aversive and negative aspects of their environment. In some individuals, they may become resigned and cease responding to environmental imperatives, even where these are inconsistent with their normal desires and goals.

In terms of the earlier parts of this chapter, much of these effects are likely to be occurring at an implicit level, without direct conscious awareness. People may not be aware of how a fear reaction has become generalized, or of how they have been impacted by chronic stress. They may not be fully aware of how, with increasing degrees of low mood, they have contracted their world and ceased to respond to their environment. We will pick these issues up again in Chapter 4 when we will look at how the brain represents and stores information, and we will come back to common client issues such as depression and anxiety in Chapters 6–8.

Points to Ponder

- If you are a practitioner or trainee, to what extent has early trauma been a significant factor in the lives of your clients?

- When you work with clients that are depressed, to what extent does it go hand in hand with anxiety?
- Thinking about typical client issues, to what extent are they "implicit" in how they operate? In other words, are clients often influenced by their experience in ways that they are not fully aware of?
- To what extent is it useful as a therapist to be aware of the biological underpinnings of mood and anxiety?

References

Abercrombie, H. C., Schaefer, S. M., Larson, C. L., Oakes, T. R., Lindgren, K. A., Holden, J. E., ... Davidson, R. J. (1998). Metabolic rate in the right amygdala predicts negative affect in depressed patients. *Neuroreport, 9*(14), 3301–3307.

Adolphs, R. (2008). Fear, faces, and the human amygdala. *Current Opinion in Neurobiology, 18*(2), 166–172.

Adolphs, R., Tranel, D., Hamann, S., Young, A. W., Calder, A. J., Phelps, E. A., ... Damasio, A. R. (1999). Recognition of facial emotion in nine individuals with bilateral amygdala damage. *Neuropsychologia, 37*(10), 1111–1117.

Anderson, J. A. (1995). *An introduction to neural networks.* Cambridge: MIT Press.

Baars, B. J. (1994). A global workspace theory of conscious experience. In A. Revonsuo & M. Kamppinen (Eds.), *Consciousness in philosophy and Cognitive neuroscience* (pp. 149–171). Hillsdale, NJ: Lawrence Erlbaum.

Baddeley, A. D. (1986). *Working memory.* Oxford: Oxford University Press.

Baddeley, A. (1992). Working memory. *Science, 255*(5044), 556–559.

Baddeley, A. (2001). The magic number and the episodic buffer. *Behavioral and Brain Sciences, 24*(1), 117–118.

Baddeley, A. D., & Hitch, G. (1974). Working memory. In G. H. Bower (Ed.), *Psychology of learning and motivation* (Vol. 8, pp. 47–89). London: Academic Press.

Bagozzi, R. P., & Pieters, R. (1998). Goal-directed emotions. *Cognition and Emotion, 12*(1), 1–26.

Baxter, J. L., Saxena, S., Brody, A. L., Ackermann, R. F., Colgan, M., Schwartz, J. M., ... Phelps, M. E. (1996, January). Brain mediation of obsessive-compulsive disorder symptoms: Evidence from functional brain imaging studies in the human and nonhuman primate. *Seminars in Clinical Neuropsychiatry, 1*(1), 32–47.

Beauregard, M., Leroux, J. M., Bergman, S., Arzoumanian, Y., Beaudoin, G., Bourgouin, P., & Stip, E. (1998). The functional neuroanatomy of major depression: An fMRI study using an emotional activation paradigm. *Neuroreport, 9*(14), 3253–3258.

Bechara, A. (2004). The role of emotion in decision-making: Evidence from neurological patients with orbitofrontal damage. *Brain and Cognition, 55*(1), 30–40.

Bruder, G. E., Stewart, J. W., Tenke, C. E., McGrath, P. J., Leite, P., Bhattacharya, N., & Quitkin, F. M. (2001). Electroencephalographic and perceptual asymmetry differences between responders and nonresponders to an SSRI antidepressant. *Biological Psychiatry, 49*(5), 416–425.

Bryant, R. A., Kemp, A. H., Felmingham, K. L., Liddell, B., Olivieri, G., Peduto, A., ... Williams, L. M. (2008). Enhanced amygdala and medial prefrontal activation during nonconscious processing of fear in posttraumatic stress disorder: An fMRI study. *Human Brain Mapping, 29*(5), 517–523.

Coffey, C. E., Wilkinson, W. E., Weiner, R. D., Djang, W. T., Webb, M. C., Figiel, G. S., & Spritzer, C. E. (1993). Quantitative cerebral anatomy in depression: A controlled magnetic resonance imaging study. *Archives of General Psychiatry, 50*(1), 7–16.

Collette, F., & Van der Linden, M. (2002). Brain imaging of the central executive component of working memory. *Neuroscience and Biobehavioral Reviews, 26*(2), 105–125.

Conway, M. A. (1990). *Autobiographical memory: An introduction*. Milton Keynes, UK: Open University Press.

Costafreda, S. G., Brammer, M. J., David, A. S., & Fu, C. H. (2008). Predictors of amygdala activation during the processing of emotional stimuli: A meta-analysis of 385 PET and fMRI studies. *Brain Research Reviews, 58*(1), 57–70.

Craik, F. I., & Tulving, E. (1975). Depth of processing and the retention of words in episodic memory. *Journal of Experimental Psychology: General, 104*(3), 268–294.

Davidson, R. J. (2000). Affective style, psychopathology, and resilience: Brain mechanisms and plasticity. *American Psychologist, 55*(11), 1196–2214.

Davidson, R. J., Pizzagalli, D., Nitschke, J. B., & Putnam, K. (2002). Depression: Perspectives from affective neuroscience. *Annual Review of Psychology, 53*(1), 545–574.

Debener, S., Beauducel, A., Nessler, D., Brocke, B., Heilemann, H., & Kayser, J. (2000). Is resting anterior EEG alpha asymmetry a trait marker for depression? *Neuropsychobiology, 41*(1), 31–37.

Dehaene, S., & Naccache, L. (2001). Towards a cognitive neuroscience of consciousness: Basic evidence and a workspace framework. *Cognition, 79*(1–2), 1–37.

De Lanerolle, N. C., Kim, J. H., Robbins, R. J., & Spencer, D. D. (1989). Hippocampal interneuron loss and plasticity in human temporal lobe epilepsy. *Brain Research, 495*(2), 387–395.

D'esposito, M., Detre, J. A., Alsop, D. C., Shin, R. K., Atlas, S., & Grossman, M. (1995). The neural basis of the central executive system of working memory. *Nature, 378*(6554), 279–285.

Dilger, S., Straube, T., Mentzel, H. J., Fitzek, C., Reichenbach, J. R., Hecht, H., … Miltner, W. H. (2003). Brain activation to phobia-related pictures in spider phobic humans: An event-related functional magnetic resonance imaging study. *Neuroscience Letters, 348*(1), 29–32.

Drevets, W. C. (2000). Functional anatomical abnormalities in limbic and prefrontal cortical structures in major depression. *Progress in Brain Research, 126*, 413–431.

Drevets, W. C. (2001). Neuroimaging and neuropathological studies of depression: Implications for the cognitive-emotional features of mood disorders. *Current Opinion in Neurobiology, 11*(2), 240–249.

Drevets, W. C., Savitz, J., & Trimble, M. (2008). The subgenual anterior cingulate cortex in mood disorders. *CNS Spectrums, 13*(8), 663–668.

Drevets, W. C., Videen, T. O., Price, J. L., Preskorn, S. H., Carmichael, S. T., & Raichle, M. E. (1992). A functional anatomical study of unipolar depression. *Journal of Neuroscience, 12*(9), 3628–3641.

Duncan, J., Burgess, P., & Emslie, H. (1995). Fluid intelligence after frontal lobe lesions. *Neuropsychologia, 33*(3), 261–268.

Ekman, P. (1992). An argument for basic emotions. *Cognition and Emotion, 6*(3–4), 169–200.

Eriksson, J., Vogel, E. K., Lansner, A., Bergström, F., & Nyberg, L. (2015). Neurocognitive architecture of working memory. *Neuron, 88*(1), 33–46.

Eysenck, M. W., & Keane, M. T. (2013). *Cognitive psychology: A student's handbook*. London: Psychology Press.

Gilbertson, M. W., Shenton, M. E., Ciszewski, A., Kasai, K., Lasko, N. B., Orr, S. P., & Pitman, R. K. (2002). Smaller hippocampal volume predicts pathologic vulnerability to psychological trauma. *Nature Neuroscience, 5*(11), 1242–1249.

Gold, J., & Stricker, G. (2001). A relational psychodynamic perspective on assimilative integration. *Journal of Psychotherapy Integration, 11*(1), 43–58.

Gould, E., Tanapat, P., Rydel, T., & Hastings, N. (2000). Regulation of hippocampal neurogenesis in adulthood. *Biological Psychiatry, 48*(8), 715–720.

Hampson, R. E., Simeral, J. D., & Deadwyler, S. A. (1999). Distribution of spatial and nonspatial information in dorsal hippocampus. *Nature, 402*(6762), 610–618.

Hasler, G., Drevets, W. C., Manji, H. K., & Charney, D. S. (2004). Discovering endophenotypes for major depression. *Neuropsychopharmacology, 29*(10), 1765–1781.

Heim, C., & Nemeroff, C. B. (2001). The role of childhood trauma in the neurobiology of mood and anxiety disorders: Preclinical and clinical studies. *Biological Psychiatry, 49*(12), 1023–1039.

Huey, E. D., Zahn, R., Krueger, F., Moll, J., Kapogiannis, D., Wassermann, E. M., & Grafman, J. (2008). A psychological and neuroanatomical model of obsessive-compulsive disorder. *The Journal of Neuropsychiatry and Clinical Neurosciences, 20*(4), 390–408.

Kim, J. J., & Diamond, D. M. (2002). The stressed hippocampus, synaptic plasticity and lost memories. *Nature Reviews Neuroscience, 3*(6), 453–461.

Lazarus, R. S. (1991). Progress on a cognitive-motivational-relational theory of emotion. *American Psychologist, 46*(8), 819–834.

Lyon, D. R., Gunzelmann, G., & Gluck, K. A. (2008). A computational model of spatial visualization capacity. *Cognitive Psychology, 57*(2), 122–152.

MacDonald, A. W., Cohen, J. D., Stenger, V. A., & Carter, C. S. (2000). Dissociating the role of the dorsolateral prefrontal and anterior cingulate cortex in cognitive control. *Science, 288*(5472), 1835–1838.

Malberg, J. E., Eisch, A. J., Nestler, E. J., & Duman, R. S. (2000). Chronic antidepressant treatment increases neurogenesis in adult rat hippocampus. *Journal of Neuroscience, 20*(24), 9104–9110.

Mayberg, H. S., Brannan, S. K., Mahurin, R. K., Jerabek, P. A., Brickman, J. S., Tekell, J. L., … Fox, P. T. (1997). Cingulate function in depression: A potential predictor of treatment response. *Neuroreport, 8*(4), 1057–1061.

Mayberg, H. S., Liotti, M., Brannan, S. K., McGinnis, S., Mahurin, R. K., Jerabek, P. A., … Fox, P. T. (1999). Reciprocal limbic-cortical function and negative mood: Converging PET findings in depression and normal sadness. *American Journal of Psychiatry, 156*(5), 675–682.

Nader, K., Schafe, G. E., & LeDoux, J. E. (2000). Fear memories require protein synthesis in the amygdala for reconsolidation after retrieval. *Nature, 406*(6797), 722–731.

Naqvi, N., Shiv, B., & Bechara, A. (2006). The role of emotion in decision making: A cognitive neuroscience perspective. *Current Directions in Psychological Science, 15*(5), 260–264.

Nutt, D. J., Ballenger, J. C., Sheehan, D., & Wittchen, H. U. (2002). Generalized anxiety disorder: Comorbidity, comparative biology and treatment. *International Journal of Neuropsychopharmacology, 5*(4), 315–325.

Paré, D., Quirk, G. J., & Ledoux, J. E. (2004). New vistas on amygdala networks in conditioned fear. *Journal of Neurophysiology, 92*(1), 1–9.

Pinel, J. P. (2013). *Biopsychology*. London: Pearson Higher Ed.

Plagnol, A. (2002). La structure pliée des espaces de représentation: théorie élémentaire. *Intellectica, 35*, 27–81.

Plagnol, A. (2004). *Espaces de représentation: Théorie élémentaire et psychopathologie* [Representational spaces: Elements and psychopathology]. Paris: Editions du CNRS.

Plagnol, A. (in press). *Principes de navigation dans les mondes possibles* [Principles of navigation in possible worlds]. Garches, France: Terra Cotta.

Ragni, M., & Knauff, M. (2013). A theory and a computational model of spatial reasoning with preferred mental models. *Psychological Review, 120*(3), 561–588.

Roca, M., Parr, A., Thompson, R., Woolgar, A., Torralva, T., Antoun, N., … Duncan, J. (2009). Executive function and fluid intelligence after frontal lobe lesions. *Brain, 133*(1), 234–247.

Rodrigues, S. M., Schafe, G. E., & LeDoux, J. E. (2004). Molecular mechanisms underlying emotional learning and memory in the lateral amygdala. *Neuron, 44*(1), 75–91.

Rumelhart, D. E. (2017). Schemata: The building blocks of cognition. In R. J. Spiro, B. C. Bruce, & W. F. Brewer (Eds.), *Theoretical issues in reading comprehension* (pp. 33–58). London: Routledge.

Sapolsky, R. M., Uno, H., Rebert, C. S., & Finch, C. E. (1990). Hippocampal damage associated with prolonged glucocorticoid exposure in primates. *Journal of Neuroscience, 10*(9), 2897–2902.

Saxena, S., Brody, A. L., Schwartz, J. M., & Baxter, L. R. (1998). Neuroimaging and frontal-subcortical circuitry in obsessive-compulsive disorder. *The British Journal of Psychiatry, 173*, 26–37.

Saxena, S., Gorbis, E., O'neill, J., Baker, S. K., Mandelkern, M. A., Maidment, K. M., ... London, E. D. (2009). Rapid effects of brief intensive cognitive-behavioral therapy on brain glucose metabolism in obsessive-compulsive disorder. *Molecular Psychiatry, 14*(2), 197–208.

Schulte-Rüther, M., Markowitsch, H. J., Fink, G. R., & Piefke, M. (2007). Mirror neuron and theory of mind mechanisms involved in face-to-face interactions: A functional magnetic resonance imaging approach to empathy. *Journal of Cognitive Neuroscience, 19*(8), 1354–1372.

Shallice, T. (1982). Specific impairments of planning. *Philosophical Transactions of the Royal Society of London. B, Biological Sciences, 298*(1089), 199–209.

Shamay-Tsoory, S. G., Aharon-Peretz, J., & Perry, D. (2009). Two systems for empathy: A double dissociation between emotional and cognitive empathy in inferior frontal gyrus versus ventromedial prefrontal lesions. *Brain, 132*(3), 617–627.

Sheline, Y. I. (2000). 3D MRI studies of neuroanatomic changes in unipolar major depression: The role of stress and medical comorbidity. *Biological Psychiatry, 48*(8), 791–800.

Sheline, Y. I., Sanghavi, M., Mintun, M. A., & Gado, M. H. (1999). Depression duration but not age predicts hippocampal volume loss in medically healthy women with recurrent major depression. *Journal of Neuroscience, 19*(12), 5034–5043.

Turner, J. C., Meyer, D. K., & Schweinle, A. (2003). The importance of emotion in theories of motivation: Empirical, methodological, and theoretical considerations from a goal theory perspective. *International Journal of Educational Research, 39*(4–5), 375–393.

3

In Search of the Good Life

1   The Motivational System

In Chapter 2, we saw that consciousness can be conceived of as a way for the brain to bring together into awareness diverse aspects of our current experience. These range from stimuli in the outside world through to complex representations of our past. Baars (1994) used the term "global workspace" to label this system. He suggested that this allows us to martial our mental resources to tackle current problems and move us towards our goals.

It was also mentioned in the previous chapter that our human motivations drive our behaviour, and that we may be more or less aware of these motives over time. One source of such motivations is our biological drives (Pinel, 2013). They can also be culturally conditioned, leading to behaviours which push us towards higher-order goals. The latter are encoded as part of the representational system, and as we will see in the next chapter, form part of our self-representational system (Conway & Pleydell-Pearce, 2000). These two sources of motivation will also interact, thus how we go about responding to our biological needs and drives will be culturally conditioned.

© The Author(s) 2019
T. Ward and A. Plagnol, *Cognitive Psychodynamics as an Integrative Framework in Counselling Psychology and Psychotherapy*,
https://doi.org/10.1007/978-3-030-25823-8_3

In terms of the biological needs and drives, these are well accepted, and much is known about how they are experienced and influence behaviour (Pinel, 2013). Thus, we have basic needs for food and water and are driven through the sexual drive to procreate and maintain the population of our species (Stein, 1989). In his very popular theory of motivation, Maslow (1943) saw such needs as these as fundamental, and clearly, humans will strive to meet these needs first. Once these are satisfied, people may move on to try and meet higher-order needs, according to a hierarchy.

As Grawe (2007) points out, there are many views within psychology as to what our basic psychological needs might be, over and above our basic biological needs. He suggests that some of the candidates put forward, such as a need for power and achievement (Brunstein & Heckhausen, 2018), should not be seen as universal. This is on the grounds that many in the population appear to get by very adequately without significant satisfaction in these domains. Grawe suggests that basic psychological needs would be such as to impact on a person's well-being and mental functioning, were they not to be fulfilled to some extent. Thus, he puts forward the suggestions of Epstein (1998, 2003) as a good candidate list, on the grounds that there is good evidence that these needs have been shown to be deeply grounded in the human nervous system by neurobiological researchers (though evidence for the fourth area is less substantial). These suggested basic needs are:

- a need for orientation, control and consistency;
- a need for pleasure and avoidance of pain;
- a need for attachment;
- a need for self-esteem enhancement.

Note that the consistency principle included in the first need is a further elaboration introduced by Grawe and not part of Epstein's original scheme. According to this principle, people strive for consistency and find inconsistency to be discomforting. So, if they have a strong need for attachment, and this is not being currently met to a satisfactory level, this will produce personal inconsistency and discomfort. This notion is compatible with Rogers' (1951) notion of incongruence,

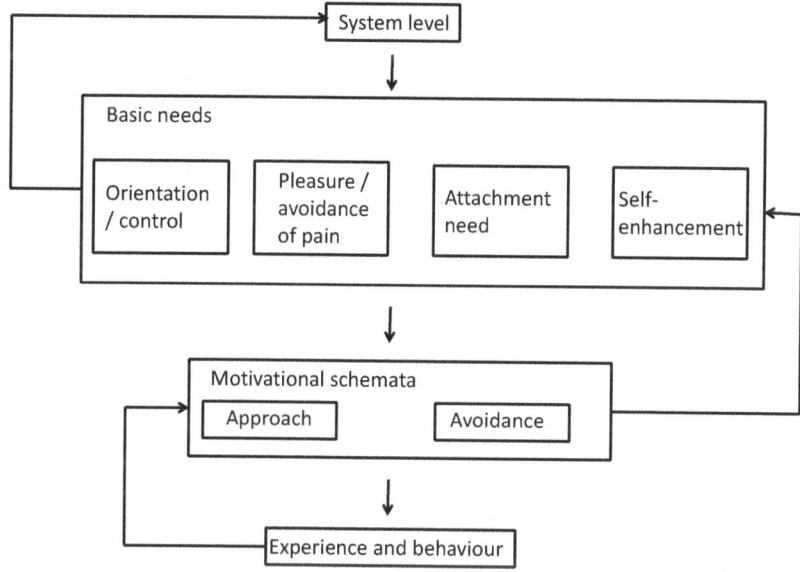

Fig. 1 The consistency theoretical model of mental functioning (After Grawe, 2007)

where someone may feel that aspects of their current self are inconsistent with their real self. An example would be where someone finds themselves in an occupation they do not really enjoy, only to realize they followed that career path to meet their parent's expectations. A diagram illustrating how these basic needs drive our behaviour and our attempts to reduce inconsistency is shown in Fig. 1.

2   Motivational Schemas and How They Operate

Looking at the lower half of Fig. 1, we can see that people try to meet their basic needs, through the deployment of motivational schemas. The term "schema" was introduced in the last chapter, to refer to organized structures within memory which can often drive behaviour in an automatic fashion. This concept will be discussed in greater depth in the next chapter, in considering in more detail how schemas organize memory and influence behaviour. For our purposes here, we can say that motivational schemas are organized units of behaviour we have developed, to help us to try and meet our basic psychological needs. The schemas which people develop are a product of their individual temperament on the one hand and the environment on the other.

These schemas can often be characterized in terms of two global tendencies, to either meet our needs through approach or avoidance tendencies. In the previous chapter, we discussed the role of emotion in cognitive control processes, and similarly, it has been proposed that there is a well-defined neural network involved in these approach/avoidance strategies (Amodio, Master, Yee, & Taylor, 2008). These are said to involve the prefrontal cortex, anterior cingulate, hippocampus and amygdala, though the two tendencies are generally conceived as two separate neural systems. These have been termed the "behavioural activation system" (BAS) and the "behavioural inhibition system" (BIS) (Gray & McNaughton, 1996). The two systems appear to operate laterally, with the BAS in the left hemisphere and the BIS on the right. Besides neuroscience research, there is also evidence to support these tendencies from personality research. Gray (1981) suggested that the BAS, associated with positive emotions, is linked to extraversion, whilst the BIS links to negative emotions and neuroticism. Both of these dimensions are represented in current theories of personality (Costa & McCrae, 1992). We saw in the previous chapter that there are patterns of reduced activation of the left prefrontal cortex and relatively stronger activation of the right prefrontal cortex in depression. Similar findings related to childhood behaviour have been found by researchers. Davidson (2013), for example, observed children at play and categorized them as inhibited or not inhibited. An EEG conducted five months later found that the inhibited children had stronger right-sided activity and vice versa for the non-inhibited. This suggests that the children with increased right-sided activation were more likely to experience negative sensations in social situations. Similarly, Davidson and Fox (1989) found that separation anxiety in infants was linked to increased right-sided activation, suggesting a greater tendency to experience negative emotion when apart from their mothers.

We all, therefore, seem to have a fairly stable tendency, which is a result of these two processes, to experience positive or negative emotions to different extents, and to react to the environment through approach or avoidance patterns. The precise balance will be unique to each individual, and for most of us, our behaviour will be a result of the interplay between the two factors. Some aspects of our behaviour will reflect an approach tendency, and others avoidance.

To help us to think about how these approach/avoidance tendencies work, it may be useful to think of some concrete examples in terms of issues which clients frequently describe. Clients who have low self-worth, perhaps as a result of frequent criticism from a parent or guardian as a child, may find it difficult to interact with other people. They expect others to judge them and consequently may avoid social contact or find social interaction a challenge. Thus, they experience anxiety in thinking about social interactions and consequently avoid situations where such interactions might be expected. In terms of their psychological needs, they are avoiding the anxiety and pain they feel in social situations. At the same time, such clients may feel extremely lonely, since like most of us they crave human warmth and connection. This draws them strongly to other people in order to meet their attachment needs. Here, we can see how, in Grawe's scheme, basic psychological needs can conflict with each other and produce conflicting approach/avoidance tendencies. Grawe termed this situation where two motivational tendencies conflict as "discordance" (as opposed to incongruence, where experience does not match desired goal states).

We will now look at each of Grawe's (2007) suggested basic needs in more detail.

3   Orientation and Control

Being able to take stock of our environment and then act upon it in a way which helps us to achieve our goals is covered by the need for orientation and control. Being successful in such endeavours will lead to positive feelings of control (Rotter, 1966) and self-efficacy (Bandura, 1997).

If we cannot achieve control, then this will be accompanied by sensations of incongruence.

In early life, the need for control will be linked to our need for attachment, as infants try to influence their mother's behaviour in response to their other basic needs such as hunger. Responsive parents will enhance the infant's feelings of control. In adulthood, the need for control may often be linked to other basic needs, such as the avoidance of pain. Where pain cannot be controlled, the discomfort and stress may be magnified. Chorpita and Barlow (1998) argued that uncontrollable threat leads to anxiety, which over time then leads to depression. This is similar to the notion of learned helplessness, where in the face of uncontrollable stress, a state of resignation and despondency is reached (Maier & Seligman, 1976).

4   Avoiding Pain/Seeking Pleasure

When we monitor the world for an event and respond to a stimulus, this causes a sequence of brain activation. This activation pattern can be picked up in the change in brain wave patterns across the surface of the scalp measured using EEG. In particular, there is a large positive amplitude that occurs 300 msecs after stimulus onset. This is called the P300 wave.

Where a stimulus is also discriminated in a negative sense, a late positive potential is produced at 650 msecs. This is most pronounced in the right hemisphere (Cacioppo, Crites, Gardner, & Berntson, 1994). Thus, the neural system is constantly responding to stimuli in our environment and coming to value judgements about them on the good vs bad continuum.

Whilst often in day-to-day life the likely evaluation of a stimulus in terms of good vs bad is obvious, for example sweet food will usually be perceived as pleasurable, this can vary depending on the context and circumstances, as well as prior learning. For example, a helping of cake will seem very unpleasant when we have just eaten a large meal and are feeling very satiated. Similarly, many foods are acquired tastes, for example children often find wine and beer to taste very unpleasant but will have changed this perception quite markedly by the time they are adults. Pleasure also does not have to be linked to direct sensory experience, for example many people may well experience pleasure from learning something new.

5   Attachment

Bowlby (1972) described how, during development, we develop an inner working model of relationships, based on our experiences with our primary caregivers. Human infants are very dependent on their caregivers in the early years of life and form attachments to these important others. Given their dependence, absence or lack of response from carers will be anxiety provoking. Over time, this interaction will lead to a basic trust or lack of it in the availability of the primary attachment figures. These early attachment relationships become encoded in implicit memory, in the same way that Young's (2014) early maladaptive schemas become encoded (see Chapter 4).

These early attachment experiences lead to the different styles and patterns of attachment which were observed by Ainsworth, Blehar, Waters, and Wall (2015). According to this work, children tended to show one of four different attachment styles. These were secure, insecure and avoidant, insecure and ambivalent, or insecure and disorganized. Two-thirds of children tend to exhibit a secure attachment style. This implies therefore that a third of children have an attachment style characterized by negative and/or avoidant emotions. These attachment patterns appear to be relatively stable (Waters, Merrick, Treboux, Crowell, & Albersheim, 2000). Changes in attachment style tended to be linked to negative life events, such as parental divorce (Beckwith, Cohen, & Hamilton, 1999).

The attachment relationship plays an important role in learning emotional containment and self-soothing (Nelson & Panksepp, 1998). When a child is hurt and in pain, the comfort of a mother, including the sounds, smells and texture lead to a release of soothing endorphins, and a rapid de-escalation of the anxiety feelings and sensations. This response is learned in the implicit memory systems, such that later a child can evoke the same reactions in self-soothing. A child without this experience will be much harder to console and will struggle to down-regulate their emotions.

Prolonged separation from attachment figures can lead to a despair reaction. Work with Rhesus monkeys shows that animals that have experienced such early separation will tend to have deeper despair reactions later (Suomi, Eisele, Grady, & Harlow, 1975).

Given the profound effects we have just described resulting from separation and poor attachment, it is perhaps not surprising that insecure attachment patterns predominate in many types of psychological distress (Cassidy & Shaver, 2002). As Grawe (2007) points out, in many conditions, such as depression, avoidance schemas around attachment may well be a predisposing factor, and not addressing these in treatment is likely to result in future recurrence.

On a positive note, developing relationships as an adult, for example as people progress from dating to marriage, tends to lead people away from insecure and disorganized attachment patterns through to more secure ones (Crowell, Treboux, & Waters, 2002). Similarly, social support and kindness can lead to positive neural growth processes (Davidson, Jackson, & Kalin, 2000).

6   Self-Esteem Enhancement

The notion that self-enhancement is a basic human motivation has been put forward by many psychologists since the advent of the discipline, including James, Mead and Cooley amongst others (Grawe, 2007).

This need seems to be one which relates mainly to humans, given that it depends upon qualities which seem to be specific to our species such as a high degree of conscious self-awareness. Furthermore, these properties develop in individuals over time. Infants are much less self-aware than adults. This human need is therefore not easily studied in young children, unlike attachment which can be disrupted from an early age.

Given the suggestion then that people strive to enhance their self-esteem, how does low self-esteem come about? Sullivan (2013) suggested that where a small child's relations with immediate caregivers are not satisfactory for some reason, the child tends to internalize this as to some extent their fault. Given the dependence on carers, Sullivan suggests that this is less anxiety provoking to the child than to see the parent as deficient.

We can, therefore, see how low self-esteem can come about. A question which arises from this is that if there is a basic drive to enhance self-esteem, why do people not work to overcome this as they get older or as adults? There seems to be a paradox here, in that people with low self-esteem often do not seem to strive to overcome this, and sometimes seem to make choices which will be detrimental rather than positive. Grawe (2007) suggests we can understand this through the complex interaction of experience on the one hand and competing psychological needs on the other. People may have grown up in an environment which has led them to expect negative outcomes despite their attempts to elicit positive responses. At the same time, there are competing demands from different psychological needs. If we strive to avoid painful experiences for example, then this may result in us sticking with avoidance schemas, so that we don't experience the negative emotion of rejection or failure. If we have been disparaged whenever we have tried to move ourselves forward, then we may prefer to keep our heads below the parapet in future.

It is also worth bearing in mind that there can be a difference between explicit self-esteem, or what people say and believe about themselves, and implicit self-esteem, which is how they actually behave and experience emotion in the world. It seems that implicit processes tend to automatically produce esteem enhancing reactions, whereas explicit processes tend to succumb to the need for consistency, such that our evaluations are consistent with current perceptions (Epstein & Morling, 1995). In therapy therefore, the better strategy to increase client self-esteem might be to engage implicit processes, by for example encouraging them to engage in positive activities which will increase their sense of personal agency.

Whilst people with low self-esteem may have an unwarrantedly negative view of themselves, it is also true that people with good self-esteem can be overly positive and have illusions about their merits.

This is true across a wide range of domains (see, e.g., review by Colvin & Block, 1994). A common illustration of this phenomenon is that most people will describe themselves as better than average drivers, whereas this cannot logically be the case for everyone! Therefore, the concern of therapists should be that clients use opportunities to enhance their self-esteem the same way that anyone else would, without worrying too much that this is realistic (except of course where people have an excessively inflated sense of their own self-worth which is in fact part of the issue they present with).

7   Defence Mechanisms as Motivational Schemas

Defence mechanisms were put forward by Anna Freud (original 1936, newer edition by Karnac, 1992) to describe the way in which the ego protects itself from uncomfortable feelings by operating on aspects of experience which would result in conflicts. The classic example is the employee who comes home from work and takes out the stress and strains of their day on the family at home, which is an example of displacement. Most therapists will recognize something similar in many of their clients, where emotions generated from their relationships with parents play out with significant others in their adult lives.

There has been debate over the years about the extent to which these defence mechanisms really are evident in people's lives in a way which can be verified objectively. One of the first interesting pieces of evidence comes from the work of Kragh (1960), who developed a subliminal threat perception test. In this test, people are shown images for very brief instances and are asked to describe what they see. Their responses are then classified in terms of the various types of defence mechanism which they are said to typify. This test has shown impressive results in terms of its ability to predict real-world outcomes. For example, it was used to look at which candidates for pilot training would go on to be successful (impressive here in the sense that correlations above 0.5 for variables which can make these kinds of predictions are rare in psychology). This work has been followed up by Cooper and Kline (1986), who suggested that the test does provide evidence for the apparent existence of a number of defence mechanisms (though they suggested the case for repression was less clear).

Researchers have also made efforts to measure these defensive styles in a more straightforward way using questionnaires (Andrews, Pollock, & Stewart, 1989; Schauenburg, Willenborg, Sammet, & Ehrenthal, 2007). The defence styles questionnaire includes such defence mechanisms as suppression, sublimation, humour, rationalization, denial, splitting, idealization, projection, displacement and reaction formation.

We would argue, in line with the motivational framework we have outlined in this chapter, that defence mechanisms are all "strategies" which people adopt to maintain consistency and reduce incongruence in relation to their basic psychological needs. Given that motivational schemas may have been acquired over many years, it is not surprising that they often operate implicitly and with little or no conscious awareness. So, for example, someone with a highly critical parent who used extreme disciplinary measures to punish failure would be very reluctant to accept blame for anything. In a situation therefore where things are not going to plan, they may habitually seek to place the fault in others and may not be consciously aware that this is taking place. This is the process of projection. Another quite common scenario might be where we are finding a new task quite difficult to master. We might explain this to ourselves as "perhaps this task does not play to my strengths, and no doubts lots of other people find this hard", i.e. a process of rationalization. Whilst many defence mechanisms seem to operate through the avoidance tendency, for example suppression or denial, others can be seen as approach oriented. For example, someone experiencing disappointment in one area of their life might compensate by expanding their energies in another, e.g. through work, a process which might be described as sublimation. The disappointment in one area of life is avoided, through approach strategies in a different area.

8   Concluding Remarks—What Are the Implications for Psychotherapy?

The first implication for therapy arising from this chapter is perhaps the observation that humans behave in a way that will help them to meet their basic psychological needs. Quite what these needs are is open to further discussion and refinement, but the four put forward by Grawe (2007), based on Epstein (1998, 2003), seem like good candidates. We know that orientation and control are very important to people, and that lack of control can lead to stress and demotivation, especially in the work environment. Avoiding pain and enhancing pleasure are consistent with our biological drives. Attachment is a need evident in early childhood, whose satisfaction or frustration has an impact on later adult relationships. Finally, most people will seek to enhance their self-esteem, though it is less clear that this principle operates consistently. It seems that it can be frustrated and neglected in some cases.

Most therapists will be able to relate these basic needs to the narratives which their clients recount in sessions. If these basic needs are frustrated then people will experience incongruence and inconsistency, and these negative feelings will potentially motivate them to seek therapy.

In trying to meet their needs, behaviour tends to be driven by two opposing tendencies, one to approach situations and one to avoid. There is a sound neurological correlate to this proposal. Such patterns will be acquired over time, so that individuals have a repertoire of motivational schemas. As with most schematic learning, these often operate at a subconscious, implicit level. The role of the therapist, therefore, is to listen to client narratives, to gain a sense of where the client's attempts to meet their basic psychological needs are being frustrated, and to listen out for the patterns of behaviour which illustrate the client's attempts to meet their needs in terms of motivational schemas. The process of therapy may increase client's insights into these patterns, so that they can avoid, moderate or adapt them. They may also then be able to appreciate where their strategies are sub-optimal and strive to develop new patterns and strategies.

Points to Ponder

- To what extent do you think most client issues are linked to basic psychological needs?
- In your experience, do client's responses to their perceived needs tend to fit within the approach versus avoidance tendencies?
- To what extent do you think it is helpful for clients to consider different ways of responding to their problems?

References

Ainsworth, M. D. S., Blehar, M. C., Waters, E., & Wall, S. N. (2015). *Patterns of attachment: A psychological study of the strange situation.* London: Psychology Press.

Amodio, D. M., Master, S. L., Yee, C. M., & Taylor, S. E. (2008). Neurocognitive components of the behavioral inhibition and activation systems: Implications for theories of self-regulation. *Psychophysiology, 45*(1), 11–19.

Andrews, G., Pollock, C., & Stewart, G. (1989). The determination of defense style by questionnaire. *Archives of General Psychiatry, 46*(5), 455–460.

Baars, B. J. (1994). A global workspace theory of conscious experience. In *Consciousness in philosophy and cognitive neuroscience* (pp. 149–171). Hillsdale: Erlbaum.

Bandura, A. (1997). *Self-efficacy: The exercise of control* (pp. 3–604). New York: W. H. Freeman.

Beckwith, L., Cohen, S. E., & Hamilton, C. E. (1999). Maternal sensitivity during infancy and subsequent life events relate to attachment representation at early adulthood. *Developmental Psychology, 35*(3), 693.

Bowlby, J. (1972). *Attachment: Attachment and loss* (Vol. 1). London: Penguin Books.

Brunstein, J. C., & Heckhausen, H. (2018). Achievement motivation. In *Motivation and action* (pp. 221–304). New York: Springer.

Cacioppo, J. T., Crites, S. L., Gardner, W. L., & Berntson, G. G. (1994). Bioelectrical echoes from evaluative categorizations: I. A late positive brain potential that varies as a function of trait negativity and extremity. *Journal of Personality and Social Psychology, 67*(1), 115–123.

Cassidy, J., & Shaver, P. R. (Eds.). (2002). *Handbook of attachment: Theory, research, and clinical applications.* London: Rough Guides.

Chorpita, B. F., & Barlow, D. H. (1998). The development of anxiety: The role of control in the early environment. *Psychological Bulletin, 124*(1), 3.

Colvin, C. R., & Block, J. (1994). Do positive illusions foster mental health? An examination of the Taylor and Brown formulation. *Psychological Bulletin, 116,* 3–20.

Conway, M. A., & Pleydell-Pearce, C. W. (2000). The construction of autobiographical memories in the self-memory system. *Psychological Review, 107*(2), 261–272.

Cooper, C., & Kline, P. (1986). An evaluation of the Defence Mechanism Test. *British Journal of Psychology, 77*(1), 19–32.

Costa, P. T., Jr., & McCrae, R. R. (1992). Four ways five factors are basic. *Personality and Individual Differences, 13*(6), 653–665.

Crowell, J. A., Treboux, D., & Waters, E. (2002). Stability of attachment representations: The transition to marriage. *Developmental Psychology, 38*(4), 467–473.

Davidson, R. J. (2013). Childhood temperament and cerebral asymmetry: A neurobiological substrate of behavioral inhibition. In *Social withdrawal, inhibition, and shyness in childhood* (pp. 41–58). London: Psychology Press.

Davidson, R. J., & Fox, N. A. (1989). Frontal brain asymmetry predicts infants' response to maternal separation. *Journal of Abnormal Psychology, 98*(2), 127–138.

Davidson, R. J., Jackson, D. C., & Kalin, N. H. (2000). Emotion, plasticity, context, and regulation: Perspectives from affective neuroscience. *Psychological Bulletin, 126*(6), 890–901.

Epstein, S. (1998). Cognitive-experiential self-theory. In *Advanced personality* (pp. 211–238). Boston, MA: Springer.

Epstein, S. (2003). Cognitive-experiential self-theory of personality. *Comprehensive Handbook of Psychology, 5,* 159–184.

Epstein, S., & Morling, B. (1995). Is the self motivated to do more than enhance and/or verify itself?. In *Efficacy, agency, and self-esteem* (pp. 9–29). Boston, MA: Springer.

Freud, A. (1992). *The ego and the mechanisms of defence.* New York: Karnac Books.

Grawe, K. (2007). *Neuropsychotherapy.* London: Psychology Press.

Gray, J. A. (1981). A critique of Eysenck's theory of personality. In *A model for personality* (pp. 246–276). Berlin, Heidelberg: Springer.

Gray, J. A., & McNaughton, N. (1996). The neuropsychology of anxiety: Reprise. In *Nebraska symposium on motivation* (Vol. 43, pp. 61–134). Lincoln: University of Nebraska Press.

Kragh, U. (1960). The Defense Mechanism Test: A new method for diagnosis and personnel selection. *Journal of Applied Psychology, 44*(5), 303.

Maier, S. F., & Seligman, M. E. (1976). Learned helplessness: Theory and evidence. *Journal of Experimental Psychology: General, 105*(1), 3–12.

Maslow, A. H. (1943). A theory of human motivation. *Psychological Review, 50*(4), 370–383.

Nelson, E. E., & Panksepp, J. (1998). Brain substrates of infant–Mother attachment: Contributions of Opioids, Oxytocin, and Norepinephrine. *Neuroscience and Biobehavioral Reviews, 22*(3), 437–452.

Pinel, J. P. (2013). *Biopsychology.* London: Pearson.

Rogers, C. R. (1951). *Client centred therapy.* London: Constable.

Rotter, J. B. (1966). Generalised expectations for internal vs external control of reinforcement. *Psychological Monographs, 80*(1), 1–28.

Schauenburg, H., Willenborg, V., Sammet, I., & Ehrenthal, J. C. (2007). Self-reported defence mechanisms as an outcome measure in psychotherapy: A study on the German version of the Defence Style Questionnaire DSQ 40. *Psychology and Psychotherapy: Theory, Research and Practice, 80*(3), 355–366.

Stein, A. (1989). Three models of sexuality: Drives, identities and practices. *Sociological Theory, 7*(1), 1–13.

Sullivan, H. S. (2013). *The interpersonal theory of psychiatry.* London: Routledge.

Suomi, S. J., Eisele, C. D., Grady, S. A., & Harlow, H. F. (1975). Depressive behavior in adult monkeys following separation from family environment. *Journal of Abnormal Psychology, 84*(5), 576–589.

Waters, E., Merrick, S., Treboux, D., Crowell, J., & Albersheim, L. (2000). Attachment security in infancy and early adulthood: A twenty-year longitudinal study. *Child Development, 71*(3), 684–689.

Young, J. E. (2014). Schema-focused therapy for personality disorders. In *Cognitive behaviour therapy* (pp. 215–236). London: Routledge.

4

Defined by Our Past

Sarah—a case of unresolved grief?
Sarah lost her brother last year. She is thirty-two years old, her brother was
thirty. He died in a car accident travelling down the motorway after going
to see some friends. The precise nature of the accident remains sketchy in
many details, though the police have tried to give the best account they can.
It seems that Simon was caught up in a multiple vehicle pileup, after a
car towing a caravan lost control in heavy winds. Sarah and Simon both
worked together for a large company. Although they worked in different
areas, their paths would cross several times a day, e.g. at the photocopier.
Sarah reports that even after a year she struggles with overwhelming sadness
and grief, and this often happens at work when she has to go to those areas
where she might bump into Simon. Other people at home have found the
loss difficult, and she has not been able to speak to her partner or parents
about it. She thinks that she should have moved on by now.

In Chapter 2, we saw that the human representational system is a major
part of the cognitive architecture, and that at any point in time only a tiny
fraction of our past experience is available to conscious experience. In this
chapter, we will explore in more detail the nature of the representational
system, and how we construct a complex and dynamic inner world.

© The Author(s) 2019
T. Ward and A. Plagnol, *Cognitive Psychodynamics as an Integrative*
Framework in Counselling Psychology and Psychotherapy,
https://doi.org/10.1007/978-3-030-25823-8_4

1   Explicit vs. Implicit Memory

There are many ways in which different aspects of memory representation have been contrasted by psychologists, and one important distinction is between implicit and explicit memory, as mentioned in previous chapters. Implicit memory refers to information which is retained by our memory processes, and which influences our subsequent behaviour and information processing, but below our level of awareness. For example, related concepts are closely linked in memory, such that the activation of one will cause related concepts to become partly active as well. Thus, if we see the word "fork", we will be quicker to recognize the word "knife" presented immediately after. This well-established phenomenon is known as *semantic priming*. In fact, all associated representations can link together in this way. If we think of a significant childhood memory (such as a favourite childhood toy), this will tend to prime and bring to mind other related memories. Our earliest memories though will often reach back to our very early childhood. As mentioned in Chapter 1, Sect. 2, for most people there is an experience of profound childhood amnesia relating to these early years (the boundary for childhood amnesia is not precisely defined, but certainly before the age of three explicit memory recall is very limited). This means that memories from this very early period are likely to be pre-verbal and experiential. We will discuss this phenomenon further shortly, along with the important concept of schemas and schematic learning.

Explicit memory refers to those memories which we can recall and verbally describe in some detail. Within these memory processes, different types of information are stored. Semantic memory refers to our knowledge of information and facts. We know, for example, that penguins are a type of flightless bird that tend to live in colder climates and eat fish which they hunt for by swimming in the sea. Episodic memory on the other hand refers to our memory for specific events and things which have happened to us. We might have specific memories, for example, of a childhood visit to a zoo, where we may have seen penguins being fed by their keeper.

2   Autobiographical Memory

From a psychotherapeutic perspective, there is an important class of explicit memory which combines both semantic and episodic aspects, and this is referred to as autobiographical memory (Conway, 1990; Conway & Pleydell-Pearce, 2000).

Figure 1 illustrates the autobiographical memory system (Conway & Pleydell-Pearce, 2000). Knowledge of the self is coded by the long-term self-system. Within the system is an autobiographical database, which includes important details about ourselves and our lives. People tend to have an overall life story, within which there may be specific periods and within these periods general events. So, we may be aware of our early childhood as one life period, and within this there may be specific memories for general events, such as family holidays. Alongside these,

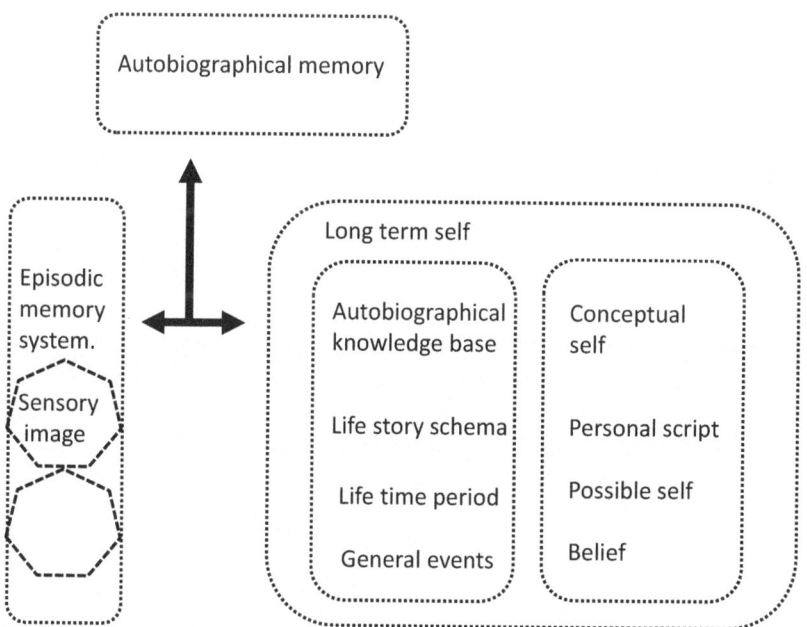

Fig. 1 The autobiographical memory system (After Conway & Pleydell-Pearce, 2000)

we have conceptual knowledge about ourselves, including information such as how we tend to go about our lives, what we think we might like to become in the future and beliefs about ourselves and others. This information, encoded in the long-term self-system, links to memories in the episodic memory system. It is this linking of specific personal memories and associated knowledge from the long-term self-system which comprises an autobiographical memory.

To bring this alive with a specific example, imagine that you are asked to remember an autobiographical memory from your early childhood. Here is a specific memory from one of us on this theme:

> In my own case, family holidays are quite prominent in this phase of my life, given that they are specific memories which tend to be different to the day to day activities going on around them during other times of the year. One specific family holiday comes to mind, perhaps because it was a particularly happy holiday, which was a summer holiday spent in the English seaside town of Great Yarmouth. This town is well known for its large amusement park on the seafront, which I recall we visited as a family on several occasions. I have a very vivid and specific memory of the snail ride, which involved sitting in the back of a large snail, as it trundled its way through an apparent underground grotto, full of various characters and displays representing well known nursery rhymes. I know from family folklore that this holiday was in 1971. I also know these snails exist to this day, as I visited them with my own daughter in 2014, as a sort of pilgrimage following my mother's death in 2013.[1]

Whilst the example above is quite specific, and possible to date to a precise year, many of our dim and distant autobiographical memories will not be as specific or as easy to pin to a given date. We may well have school-based memories, for example, of particular classrooms, teachers, specific lessons and so on, but we may struggle to pin these to a precise chronology.

According to Conway, there is a part of the self-memory system which remains active in the present moment and which influences our

---

[1]This is a reminiscence from TW.

behaviour, perceptions and memory. This is the *working self*, an important aspect of which is representing our current and long-term goals. As we noted in the earlier chapter on cognitive neuroscience, there is evidence for a cognitive affective system in the frontal parts of the brain (Davidson, Pizzagalli, Nitschke, & Putnam, 2002) which processes approach and avoidance goals. There is therefore a link between the self-memory system, our motivation, goals and priorities, and our memory processing and retention.

3 Self-defining Memories

Some autobiographical memories have been noted to be particularly vivid and intense. They may include affective aspects, be frequently rehearsed and link to other similar memories. They may be linked to certain concerns or unresolved conflicts. These vivid recollections have been termed *self-defining memories* (SDMs) and can be differentiated from other vivid memories such as flashbulb memory (Pillemer, 2009). According to Conway (1990), SDMs can be differentiated from other memories by the fact that they link to themes which are part of the narrative account of the individual, and that they relate to concerns or unresolved conflicts. The narrative themes will typically involve goals from the working self-construct construct.

According to Conway and Pleydell-Pearce (2000), goals within the working self will reflect important developmental objectives such as growth, autonomy, achievement, intimacy, generativity, ageing, loss and the associated existential issues. Frequently SDMs will be implicated in core individual goals (Moffitt & Singer, 1994). Where these goals are changing, and where the degree of discrepancy is large, greater degrees of affect will be experienced, leading to increased generation of SDMs. Given this, it seems highly likely that SDMs will be a frequent subject of discussion and reflection in psychotherapy. This seems to be the case. Singer and colleagues have shown across a number of studies (e.g. Singer & Blagov, 2004; Singer & Salovey, 1996) that SDMs are linked to important relational themes that play out in clients interpersonal relationships, as well as in the transference observed during the therapeutic process (see later in this chapter for further discussion of transference from an implicit memory perspective). Furthermore, SDMs can play a role in mood regulation. For example, non-depressed individuals may use positive SDMs to counter negative mood states, whilst depressed individuals are less likely to employ this strategy (Josephson, 1996). Similarly, Moffitt and Singer (1994) found that depressed individuals were less likely to recall specific SDMs when asked to recall a positive memory but did not differ from controls in terms of negative memory recall.

4   Explicit Memory and Psychotherapy

As we have seen, self-defining memories often relate to the core goals of an individual. In the previous chapter on motivation, we saw that core goals tend to focus on a small number of key psychological needs, such as the need to reduce pain and enhance control. We also saw how people tend to use either approach or avoidance tendencies in trying to meet their goals, and that at any one time the degree to which people feel they are meeting their goals will be linked to a feeling of congruence. Where people are failing to meet their goals, there will be a strong degree of incongruence between actuality and their desired goal states, leading to a strong sense of discomfort. This internal sense of incongruence is what leads many clients to seek therapy, and in examining their psychological distress, self-defining memories are likely to play a big role in their narrative. We also noted in the previous chapter that people's strategies for achieving goals become schematized, that is they enact a routine behavioural repertoire, often with little consciousawareness. For example, someone that fears social situations may routinely avoid instances where they think there might be a lot of people present, though they may be unaware that this is what they are doing at the time.

As we have seen in Chapter 3, Sect. 5, one of the core basic psychological needs is around attachment, the need to be in relationship with other people. According to Bowlby (1972), people develop internal working models of relationship (IWMs), which typically result from people's interaction with significant others during childhood. These IWMs will impact on people's later adult relationships. The adult attachment interview (George, Kaplan, & Main, 1985) allows the style of adult relationship to be categorized into three themes. In the first, secure autonomous, people have a coherent childhood narrative and can freely recall specific aspects and memories. In the preoccupied or entangled style, people have a preoccupied, angry or confused relationship with their carers. In the dismissing style, people have a tendency to dismiss or draw attention away from negative or unfavourable childhood experiences. As Conway, Singer, and Tagini (2004) note, these attachment styles will be reflected in the nature and content of the SDMs which people recall. Given that the last two styles may well be associated with difficulties in adult relationships, they may well again feature strongly in the narratives recounted by clients in sessions with therapists. Given the importance of early childhood experience in determining our relational patterns, specific SDMs may come from these early years. However, peoples' explicit memory for early life can be very patchy (see the later section on infantile amnesia). In our experience therefore, vivid SDMs are often highly representative of the general environment and context. Consider the narrative, for example, of a client who was abandoned on a shopping trip by his mother, having become separated from her in a busy market place. This event may have turned out well in a sense that the client was able to find their way home, but the event itself may be representative of many instances where the client felt that the mother did not look out for their wellbeing.

As with other schematic patterns of behaviour which people develop in their goal-seeking repertoire, people will frequently be unaware of how their IWMs play out in their adult relationships, or indeed in the relationship with their therapist. Such phenomena show the impact and relevance of implicit memory in psychotherapy. Whilst explicit memory and SDMs could be seen as phenomena which play out within the conscious realm of the theatre of the mind, implicit memory can be seen as exerting its influence behind the scenes, out of conscious awareness. With regard to the theatre of the mind metaphor (Baars, 1997), implicit memory could be seen as impacting on everything which happens outside of the central focus of the stage, e.g. the lighting, the props, the scenery, what play is to be performed, how the actors will portray their parts, etc. This is the subject of the next section.

5   Implicit Memory and Schemas

"Implicit memory" is the term used to describe situations where past experience and learning can be demonstrated to have an impact on current behaviour, but this takes place outside of direct consciousawareness. The example was given earlier of semantic priming, where one word, e.g. "dog", is recognized more quickly when preceded by a related word such as "cat". This phenomenon has been a leading paradigm within cognitive research on memory and language, now supported by many thousands of studies (Eysenck & Keane, 2013). It is generally ascribed to the way memory is structured and especially involves the notion of schemas.

5.1   Schemas

According to Johnson and Hasher (1987), it was Kant (1929) who first outlined the view that our previous experience and representations of the world drive our current perception and sense-making. In early psychological research, Bartlett (1932) conducted an experiment in which people had to remember a novel story, written in such a way that it did not easily fit within their current conceptions. The story was a Native American story called "war of the ghosts". It was evident from the remembered versions that people had altered the details as they listened, so that these fitted with their familiar ideas and models of the world.

In the 1970s, theories were advanced to account for phenomena evident in semantic memory, such as language priming effects. It was suggested (Collins & Loftus, 1975; Collins & Quillian, 1970) that information is organized in hierarchical structures of associated memories (see Fig. 2). Such structures can account for observed phenomena such as priming, or length of time to make decisions about knowledge statements (e.g. "cats have whiskers"). Extended networks of related information came to be termed "schemas", a concept widely applied to education and reading (Anderson, 1984). In reading, for example, it is suggested that as we read a sentence, our knowledge is activated along with associated concepts as well our knowledge of normal language patterns, such that the next word in sequence is activated almost automatically.

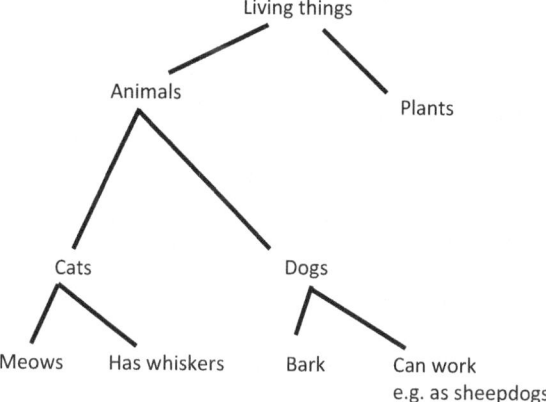

Fig. 2 The hierarchical associative conceptual system

5.2 Application of Schema Theory to Therapy

Rumelhart (1980) put forward a much more general view of memory schemas, suggesting, for example, that knowledge of ourselves is stored in these structures (corresponding to Conway and Pleydell-Pearce's [2000] long-term self). All kinds of information about ourselves may be stored, including, for example, our attitudes and confidence around subjects such as maths (Karsenty, 2004), or our appearance (Ledoux, Winterowd, Richardson, & Clark, 2010).

Rumelhart, McClelland, and PDP Research Group (1988) went on to show how such knowledge structures and schemas can be modelled using artificial intelligence. Their approach uses simplified artificial neurons, connected together in layers. The models are trained to represent information by presenting them with input and output patterns, and tweaking the links between the neurons gradually. Eventually, when shown a given input pattern, the network will produce the required output. This uses a software algorithm known as "back propagation".

Artificial neural networks have been shown to be extremely powerful. They are behind most complex artificial intelligence, including such things as predictive text, language translation and voice recognition. Such models have intriguing properties. Tryon (2014) has described in depth how such models may help us to think about human representation and psychotherapy.

To begin with, Tryon makes the point that schematic, implicit memory processes can be seen as unconscious. This suggests that a considerable amount of human information processing occurs without awareness, including the initial stage of learning. Secondly, he points out that such models are exquisite pattern completers. If a partial pattern is presented, the model will be able to make up for the missing information and predict the required output. Thus, such models have strong powers of generalization. This has implications for therapy. For example, it suggests that if we learn to associate anxiety with a particular situation, other situations which resemble the original situation to some degree will also trigger anxiety. This is at a level below consciousawareness.

Young, Klosko, and Weishaar (2003) have extended these ideas around schemas into a system of therapy, called "schema therapy". This is based on the notion that people acquire, through their developmental experience, set ways of relating to other people. Certain developmental experiences can give rise to patterns of memory and behaviour, based on past relations and emotions, which lead to maladaptive patterns in adult life. Consider, for example, the situation where someone experienced as a child often being placed in an adult role, perhaps because their carers themselves were in need of care. In such circumstances, they may become parentified. This can manifest itself in adult life as a need to look out for and care for other people, to the detriment of meeting one's own needs.

Young et al. (2003) have identified a number of such schematic patterns (18 at the time of writing—see list below). This approach to therapy has been found to be helpful for a number of conditions, including resistant depression and personality disorder (Young, 2014). Clients with conditions which frequently present in psychotherapy such as anxiety and depression typically will show evidence of a number of early maladaptive schemas. This provides possible evidence of the role of early experience in the genesis of such conditions (Calvete, Orue, & Hankin, 2013; Harris & Curtin, 2002).

Young's 18 maladaptive schemas are:

1. Abandonment/Instability (AB)
2. Mistrust/Abuse (MA)

3. Emotional deprivation (ED)
4. Defectiveness/Shame (DS)
5. Social isolation/Alienation (SI)
6. Dependence/Incompetence (DI)
7. Vulnerability to harm or illness (VH)
8. Enmeshment/Undeveloped self (EM)
9. Failure to achieve (FA)
10. Entitlement/Grandiosity (ET)
11. Insufficient self-control/Self-discipline (IS)
12. Subjugation (SP)
13. Self-sacrifice (SS)
14. Approval-seeking/Recognition-seeking (AS)
15. Negativity/Pessimism (NP)
16. Emotional Inhibition (EI)
17. Unrelenting Standards/Hypercriticalness (US)
18. Punitiveness (PU)

There is now a wealth of literature showing that schematic representations are implicated in a range of mental health conditions. Much of this concerns self-schemas. For example, in terms of general vulnerability to psychopathology, Kelvin, Goodyer, Teasdale, and Brechin (1999) found that adolescents with negative self-schemas were at increased risk. In relation to specific conditions, evidence has been found for a role for schemas in borderline personality disorder[2] (Barazandeh, Kissane, Saeedi, & Gordon, 2016), bipolar depression (Nilsson, Jørgensen, Straarup, & Licht, 2010), eating disorders (Trottier, McFarlane, & Olmsted, 2013), and social phobia and panic (Van Niekerk, Moller, & Nortje, 1999). In relation to psychosis, Appiah-Kusi et al. (2017) found evidence for schematic representations of childhood trauma. There is also evidence for schematic representations in paranoia (Tiernan, Tracey, & Shannon, 2014), persecutory delusions (Kesting & Lincoln, 2013) and delusional

---

[2]We use the terms here, and throughout the book, which were given in the original research reports. We do not condone such terms and would normally seek to use non-pathologizing descriptions.

beliefs more generally (Vázquez, Diez-Alegría, Hernández-Lloreda, & Moreno, 2008). There is considerable work on depression. Segal suggested in 1988 that negative self-schemas played a role in this condition. Dentale et al. (2016) showed a role for automatic negative self-schema activation, whilst Asarnow, Thompson, Joormann, and Gotlib (2014) suggested that negative self-schemas were a characteristic of children at risk for the condition. We will review the extensive evidence in relation to depression in the later chapter dedicated to this condition.

To summarize this section, there is now considerable evidence that implicit schematic memory processes are involved in many mental health conditions. Whether these schemas fall into those described by Young et al. (2003), or reflect our representations about ourselves more generally, they will impact upon on our interactions with others, and our ongoing mood states.

6   Childhood Amnesia

As mentioned above, a phenomenon of explicit memory is that adults do not remember very much from the very early years of their life, in effect from before the age of about four years old. There are different views about why this is (see Bauer, 2015, for a recent and rich discussion). Perner and Ruffman (1995) suggest that it is because children only develop the ability to remember events as things they have experienced between the ages of three and six years. Fivush, Haden, and Adam (1995) suggest that pre-schoolers narratives about self will develop more structure and coherence over time (though they also noted that even the youngest children had some degree of self-narrative). In terms of the age boundaries of infantile amnesia, Usher and Neisser (1993) suggest that some memories are evident from the age of two to three years. Peterson, Grant, and Boland (2005) found that children between the ages of six and nine are able to access some very early memories (with an average age of earliest recollection of thirty-nine months, but with some individuals recalling much earlier events, with the earliest being approximately nineteen months).

Whatever the precise nature and basis of infantile amnesia, the key point is that adults have very little recall of events from their very earliest years, though that is not to say there might not be fleeting memories of a small number of discrete events. However, this does not mean that there is no significant schematic learning from this early period, and the nature of implicit learning is such that this may be difficult to verbalize (James, Southam, & Blackburn, 2004). The consequence for someone whose early environment was anxiety provoking is that they may have learned to experience anxiety in relation to a number of stimuli but may not be aware of this tendency as adults. As Bonanno (1990) suggests, representations are complex and consist of a variety of different types of information, which may not always lend themselves to linguistic expression. Therapists therefore need to be aware of this, and open to helping clients to explore all aspects of their memory and experience, including bodily and sensory sensations.

7   Schemas and Transference

Transference is the process whereby patterns of behaviour we have developed over time, from our interactions with key individuals, come to be activated and thus "transferred" onto our interactions with new, unrelated, individuals (Huprich, 2010; Lemma, 2003).

As we have seen above, schematic memory can involve aspects of our self-knowledge, as well as our relationships with other people (Rumelhart, 1980; Young et al., 2003). Thus, our social interactions in part shape aspects of our self-structure (Andersen, Chen, & Miranda, 2002). When we are with new people we have not previously met, our past relational learning may be triggered, and this activation may bring with it affective aspects (Andersen & Baum, 1994; Baum & Andersen, 1999). Given the principles of implicit memory (Tryon, 2014), the precise nature of the stimulus which triggers such activation could be many and varied. It might the tone of somebody's voice, their mannerisms, or the way they structure their conversation. Furthermore, people are likely to be completely unaware of this process going on.

Our working self-concept (Conway & Playdell-Pearce, 2000) will shift as a consequence, so that the active concepts resemble those that have been acquired through the interactions we have had with the particular significant other. To illustrate this, imagine that we had a very critical parent as a child, and that in their presence we tend to feel inadequate and incompetent. As an adult, a stranger may, through asking a question in a certain way, reactivate our schemas of interactions with the critical parent. This then leads us to feel inadequate and incompetent with the stranger. We may be puzzled by this occurrence but remain completely unaware of why this has happened or come about.

This has therapeutic implications, in that interactions with a therapist could well lead a client to experience activations of learned patterns from their interactions with significant others (Andersen & Miranda, 2007). There are also implications for clinical conditions, in that these patterns of activation might be linked to low mood and self-esteem, and feelings of rejection within the working self-concept (Miranda, Andersen, & Edwards, 2013).

8   Concluding Remarks—The Implications of Memory Theory for Psychotherapy

To summarize what we have covered in this chapter, psychologists make various distinctions in relation to memory, an important one of which is the divide between implicit and explicit processes. In terms of explicit memories, people tend to have the richest and most elaborate memories about themselves. Conway et al. (2004) have outlined how different types of information are integrated in the autobiographical memory system. These authors suggest that there are well-formed memories, which often relate to our needs and goals and involve strong emotional states. These are referred to as "self-defining memories", and it is these which are likely to be the focus of much of the discussion which takes place in therapy.

At the same time, much of our past learning and memory is encoded implicitly, and as such is less open to introspection and verbalization. This can impact in important ways on much of our behaviour, for example, in terms of what we choose to attend to, and which choices we make about how we live our lives and move forward. As we have seen in the above section, such implicit patterns may well have a strong role to play in how we perceive and react to other people, and this may be an important dimension in therapy. Traditionally, this tendency to react to other people based on previous relational patterns has been called "transference" and "countertransference". The strength of this will vary from one client to another. For some clients, where previous relationships have made a big impact, there may be a strong tendency to react to others based on these previous experiences, and this may be a significant aspect of the therapy. For other clients, this may be much less the case, and other client concerns may well be more prominent.

We will end this chapter by coming back to the client vignette we started with, Sarah, a possible case of complex grief.

After several sessions with Sarah, it was evident that she had found the loss of her brother to be deeply distressing. As is often the case, some of the discussion was around society's apparent norms around grieving, and the difficulty Sarah had in being able to talk to someone about the loss. It is also common in such cases that relatives feel that they need to know as much about what happened as possible, as if the brain won't allow the person to move on until all aspects of the event have been accounted for. In relation to her day to day routine, Sarah found it extremely difficult as she moved about the office, as she had associated certain parts of the building with her brother. This was especially the case when she had to use the photocopier. Sarah was very troubled by the extreme feelings of sadness and loss which came over her at these times, and she felt that some months on from the accident she ought to have moved on. She felt as though there must be something wrong that she would still be finding this difficult after such a period of time.

Sarah found it very helpful when it was explained that the brain forms strong schematic memories and associations. As a result, it is not surprising that when she goes to parts of the office where she may have encountered Simon, she will be quite likely to think of him. The fact that the sense of loss is profound reflects the strength of Sarah's attachment and closeness to Simon. It is not unusual or a sign of something being wrong, for people to find it difficult to move on from such a loss and for it to take some considerable time. Sarah found these perspectives to be very helpful, and ended the therapy after fourteen sessions.

Points to Ponder

- If you think of particular strong memories you have from childhood, to what extent do these fit in with the notion of self-defining memories? Are they related to basic psychological needs and is there a strong emotional component?
- What is the earliest memory you can recall? Are you able to verify this memory? Was it, for example, confirmed by a parent?
- What schematic learning around relationships did you acquire as a child? Do you generally feel trusting and secure with other people? Do you sometimes suspect other people's motives? Are there certain people you feel less secure with? Why might this be? How do you relate to people who have power over you, at work for example?

References

Anderson, R. C. (1984). Some reflections on the acquisition of knowledge. *Educational Researcher, 13*(9), 5–10.

Andersen, S. M., & Baum, A. (1994). Transference in interpersonal relations: Inferences and affect based on significant-other representations. *Journal of Personality, 62*(4), 459–497.

Andersen, S. M., Chen, S., & Miranda, R. (2002). Significant others and the self. *Self and Identity, 1*(2), 159–168.

Andersen, S. M., & Miranda, R. (2007). The therapeutic relationship: Implications from social cognition and transference. In *The therapeutic relationship in the cognitive behavioral psychotherapies* (pp. 79–105). London: Routledge.

Appiah-Kusi, E., Fisher, H. L., Petros, N., Wilson, R., Mondelli, V., Garety, P. A., … Bhattacharyya, S. (2017). Do cognitive schema mediate the association between childhood trauma and being at ultra-high risk for psychosis? *Journal of Psychiatric Research, 88,* 89–96.

Asarnow, L. D., Thompson, R. J., Joormann, J., & Gotlib, I. H. (2014). Children at risk for depression: Memory biases, self-schemas, and genotypic variation. *Journal of Affective Disorders, 159,* 66–72.

Baars, B. J. (1997). In the theatre of consciousness: Global workspace theory, a rigorous scientific theory of consciousness. *Journal of Consciousness Studies, 4*(4), 292–309.

Barazandeh, H., Kissane, D. W., Saeedi, N., & Gordon, M. (2016). A systematic review of the relationship between early maladaptive schemas and borderline personality disorder/traits. *Personality and Individual Differences, 94,* 130–139.

Bartlett, F. C. (1932). *Remembering: An experimental and social study.* Cambridge: Cambridge University.

Bauer, P. J. (2015). A complementary process account of the development of childhood amnesia and a personal past. *Psychological Review, 122*(2), 204–231.

Baum, A., & Andersen, S. M. (1999). Interpersonal roles in transference: Transient mood effects under the condition of significant-other resemblance. *Social Cognition, 17*(2), 161–185.

Bonanno, G. A. (1990). Remembering and psychotherapy. *Psychotherapy: Theory, Research, Practice, Training, 27*(2), 175.

Bowlby, J. (1972). *Attachment: Attachment and loss* (Vol. 1). London: Penguin Books.

Calvete, E., Orue, I., & Hankin, B. L. (2013). Early maladaptive schemas and social anxiety in adolescents: The mediating role of anxious automatic thoughts. *Journal of Anxiety Disorders, 27*(3), 278–288.

Collins, A. M., & Loftus, E. F. (1975). A spreading-activation theory of semantic processing. *Psychological Review, 82*(6), 407–418.

Collins, A. M., & Quillian, M. R. (1970). Does category size affect categorization time? *Journal of Verbal Learning and Verbal Behavior, 9*(4), 432–438.

Conway, M. A. (1990). *Autobiographical memory: An introduction.* Milton Keynes: Open University Press.

Conway, M. A., & Pleydell-Pearce, C. W. (2000). The construction of autobiographical memories in the self-memory system. *Psychological Review, 107*(2), 261.

Conway, M. A., Singer, J. A., & Tagini, A. (2004). The self and autobiographical memory: Correspondence and coherence [Special issue]. *Social Cognition, 22*(5), 491–529.

Davidson, R. J., Pizzagalli, D., Nitschke, J. B., & Putnam, K. (2002). Depression: Perspectives from affective neuroscience. *Annual Review of Psychology, 53*(1), 545–574.

Dentale, F., Grano, C., Muzi, M., Pompili, M., Erbuto, D., & Violani, C. (2016). Measuring the automatic negative self-schema: New evidence for the construct and criterion validity of the Depression Implicit Association. *Self and Identity, 15*(5), 599–613.

Eysenck, M. W., & Keane, M. T. (2013). *Cognitive psychology: A student's handbook*. London: Psychology Press.

Fivush, R., Haden, C., & Adam, S. (1995). Structure and coherence of preschoolers' personal narratives over time: Implications for childhood amnesia. *Journal of Experimental Child Psychology, 60*(1), 32–56.

George, C., Kaplan, N., & Main, M. (1985). *The adult attachment interview*. Berkeley, CA: University of California.

Harris, A. E., & Curtin, L. (2002). Parental perceptions, early maladaptive schemas, and depressive symptoms in young adults. *Cognitive Therapy and Research, 26*(3), 405–416.

Huprich, S. K. (2010). *Psychodynamic therapy: Conceptual and empirical foundations*. London: Routledge.

James, I. A., Southam, L., & Blackburn, I. M. (2004). Schemas revisited. *Clinical Psychology and Psychotherapy, 11*(6), 369–377.

Johnson, M. K., & Hasher, L. (1987). Human learning and memory. *Annual Review of Psychology, 38*(1), 631–668.

Josephson, B. R. (1996). Mood regulation and memory: Repairing sad moods with happy memories. *Cognition and Emotion, 10*(4), 437–444.

Kant, I. (1929). *Critique of pure reason* (N. K. Smith, Trans.). New York, NY: St. Marin's Press. (Original work published in 1781 and 1787).

Karsenty, R. (2004). Mathematical self-schema: A framework for analyzing adults' retrospection on high school mathematics. *The Journal of Mathematical Behavior, 23*(3), 325–349.

Kelvin, R. G., Goodyer, I. M., Teasdale, J. D., & Brechin, D. (1999). Latent negative self-schema and high emotionality in well adolescents at risk for psychopathology. *The Journal of Child Psychology and Psychiatry and Allied Disciplines, 40*(6), 959–968.

Kesting, M. L., & Lincoln, T. M. (2013). The relevance of self-esteem and self-schemas to persecutory delusions: A systematic review. *Comprehensive Psychiatry, 54*(7), 766–789.

Ledoux, T., Winterowd, C., Richardson, T., & Clark, J. D. (2010). Relationship of negative self-schemas and attachment styles with appearance schemas. *Body Image, 7*(3), 213–217.

Lemma, A. (2003). *Introduction to the practice of psychoanalytic psychotherapy.* Chichester: Wiley.

Miranda, R., Andersen, S. M., & Edwards, T. (2013). The relational self and pre-existing depression: Implicit activation of significant-other representations exacerbates dysphoria and evokes rejection in the working self-concept. *Self and Identity, 12*(1), 39–57.

Moffitt, K. H., & Singer, J. A. (1994). Continuity in the life story: Self-defining memories, affect, and approach/avoidance personal strivings. *Journal of Personality, 62*(1), 21–43.

Nilsson, A. K. K., Jørgensen, C. R., Straarup, K. N., & Licht, R. W. (2010). Severity of affective temperament and maladaptive self-schemas differentiate borderline patients, bipolar patients, and controls. *Comprehensive Psychiatry, 51*(5), 486–491.

Perner, J., & Ruffman, T. (1995). Episodic memory and autonoetic conciousness: Developmental evidence and a theory of childhood amnesia. *Journal of Experimental Child Psychology, 59*(3), 516–548.

Peterson, C., Grant, V., & Boland, L. (2005). Childhood amnesia in children and adolescents: Their earliest memories. *Memory, 13*(6), 622–637.

Pillemer, D. B. (2009). *Momentous events, vivid memories.* Cambridge, MA: Harvard University Press.

Rumelhart, D. E. (1980). Schemata: The building blocks of cognition. In R. J. Spiro, et al. (Eds.), *Theoretical issues in reading comprehension.* Hillsdale, NJ: Lawrence Erlbaum.

Rumelhart, D. E., McClelland, J. L., & PDP Research Group. (1988). *Parallel distributed processing* (Vol. 1, p. 184). Cambridge: MIT press.

Segal, Z. V. (1988). Appraisal of the self-schema construct in cognitive models of depression. *Psychological Bulletin, 103*(2), 147–159.

Singer, J. A., & Blagov, P. S. (2004). Self-defining memories, narrative identity, and psychotherapy. In L. E. Angus & J. McLeod (Eds.), *The handbook of narrative and psychotherapy: Practice, theory and research* (pp. 229–338). Thousand Oaks, CA: Sage.

Singer, J. A., & Salovey, P. (1996). Motivated memory: Self-defining memories, goals, and affect regulation. In L. L. Martin & A. Tesser (Eds.), *Striving and feeling: Interactions among goals, affect, and self-regulation* (pp. 229–250). Mahwah, NJ: Erlbaum Associates.

Tiernan, B., Tracey, R., & Shannon, C. (2014). Paranoia and self-concepts in psychosis: A systematic review of the literature. *Psychiatry Research, 216*(3), 303–313.

Trottier, K., McFarlane, T., & Olmsted, M. P. (2013). A test of the weight-based self-evaluation schema in eating disorders: Understanding the link between self-esteem, weight-based self-evaluation, and body dissatisfaction. *Cognitive Therapy and Research, 37*(1), 122–126.

Tryon, W. (2014). *Cognitive neuroscience and psychotherapy: Network principles for a unified theory.* London: Academic Press.

Usher, J. A., & Neisser, U. (1993). Childhood amnesia and the beginnings of memory for four early life events. *Journal of Experimental Psychology: General, 122*(2), 155–166.

Van Niekerk, J. K., Möller, A. T., & Nortje, C. (1999). Self-schemas in social phobia and panic disorder. *Psychological Reports, 84*(3), 843–854.

Vázquez, C., Diez-Alegría, C., Hernández-Lloreda, M. J., & Moreno, M. N. (2008). Implicit and explicit self-schema in active deluded, remitted deluded, and depressed patients. *Journal of Behavior Therapy and Experimental Psychiatry, 39*(4), 587–599.

Young, J. E. (2014). Schema-focused therapy for personality disorders. In *Cognitive behaviour therapy* (pp. 215–236). London: Routledge.

Young, J. E., Klosko, J. S., & Weishaar, M. E. (2003). *Schema therapy: A practitioner's guide.* New York: Guilford Press.

5

Principles of Cognitive Psychodynamic Therapy

Hilary

Hilary was a 23 year old female client who presented to therapy complaining that she did not feel satisfied with her everyday relationships, and she did not know why. She knew that she was often left feeling frustrated after interactions with her relatives and friends. She had attended counselling previously some years before, following a trauma as a young teenager, after she was physically assaulted by a friend of her mother. At that point she had been living with her mother following her parent's divorce. She felt her mother had not taken the assault seriously enough, which had left her feeling very confused. At this point though, she felt she had put this behind her, and her reason for attending counselling at this time was her feeling that there was something that was making her day to day relationships difficult.

In Chapter 1, we reviewed the main perspectives that are currently evident within the realm of psychotherapy. In thinking about these various approaches, we also discussed what an effective and convincing theory of therapy needs to cover. It was suggested that an effective approach needs to provide a rich and detailed account of human experience and development (Lapworth & Sills, 2010). It would also need to be able to account for how people relate to each other, including within the

© The Author(s) 2019
T. Ward and A. Plagnol, *Cognitive Psychodynamics as an Integrative Framework in Counselling Psychology and Psychotherapy,*
https://doi.org/10.1007/978-3-030-25823-8_5

therapeutic context. Finally, it would need to be able to account for the process of therapy, in terms of what makes it effective and how clients are able to use the experience to change and move forwards in their lives (as reflected by Cooper, 2019, all therapeutic approaches have a common theme in terms of clients seeking positive movement in their lives).

In the subsequent chapters, we have then gone on to review what the psychological and cognitive science literature has to tell us about human experience and development. We have sought to frame this in terms of how it might usefully inform and help us to develop psychotherapy. In Chapter 2, we looked at the neuroscience, and what we currently know about human cognitive phenomenology, and the roles of emotions such as anxiety in thought and decision-making. In Chapter 3, we went on to look at human motivation, and the various basic psychological needs which have been suggested as fundamental to human striving and needs for achievement. In Chapter 4, we looked in more detail at how the human brain retains and represents information. We noted that whilst much of our past experience is open to conscious recollection, especially vivid self-defining memories, much of our past is retained as behavioural patterns and repertories. This latter aspect is one which we are frequently much less aware off, and which we may struggle to verbalize.

1 Findings from the Literature Which Guide Cognitive Psychodynamic Therapy

Given this review of the psychological literature, we are now therefore in a position to summarize key points about the nature of human experience and phenomenology, as follows:

– People build up complex internal representations of their experiences and the world.
– Early experiences may be in an experiential, nonverbal form.
– These representations can include behavioural repertoires/scripts. These may have built up over an extended period of time, for example, ways of feeling/reacting in relationships. People may be unaware of this and may find these aspects difficult to articulate.

- Those representations which concern the self are the most elaborate and include life narratives and goals.
- Conscious awareness is influenced and directed by these internal representations, and people are often unaware of these subtle biases.
- Much of our past experience and mental representations remain outside of conscious awareness for much of the time.
- People strive to meet their basic psychological needs.
- This striving is driven by two basic behaviour systems, one around avoidance (of things like painful stimuli), the other around approach (of rewarding and positive experiences).
- This striving process is also directed by representational schemas and scripts. Some of these could be conceived as underlying traditional defence mechanisms, for example, someone may avoid social situations if this makes them anxious but rationalize that they don't really like social events anyway. This avoids the anxiety but does not meet their attachment needs.
- If people fail to move towards meeting their basic psychological needs and goals, this will lead to psychological discomfort. More generally, *lack of internal consistency or incongruence will lead to internal tension.*
- Behaviour is both external and internal, such that psychological processes will impact on how people go about navigating their external space *but also and above all their internal space (their inner world)*. For example, people with depression have a tendency, of which they may be largely unaware, to cut down on the representational space they access. This may be due to the negative memories which they have experienced as unpleasant in the past.

Given this view of human experience and phenomenology, we can then go on to suggest the following principles as a guide. Cognitive psychodynamic therapy should therefore:

- Recognize that *every client has a complex inner world*, resulting from their individual lived experience.
- Acknowledge the insights for any one client will be unique to them.

- Be flexible in terms of time—some clients will gain useful insights quickly, others will need much more time, as the patterns to be explored may be subtle.
- Give space to clients to verbalize their concerns, and feelings of incongruence and inconsistency.
- Recognize that for many clients the nature of the incongruence/difficulties will be difficult to verbalize.
- Recognize and explore the schemas/patterns which may be driving the client's behaviour/incongruence.
- Use the therapeutic relationship as one avenue in which the client's schematic ways of relating will play out—but also recognizing that the therapist may not trigger particular issues/patterns.
- Recognize that the therapeutic relationship and space are also a venue for clients to experience new ways of relating and build new schematic patterns which can guide future behaviour.
- Offer interpretations as far as possible in a tentative fashion, *from the client's frame of reference*, so that they do not get enmeshed in the client's relational schemas.
- Enable clients to become aware of their behavioural schemas and scripts, so that they can intervene and choose to do things differently.
- Help clients to develop new schemas/scripts, so that they can successfully change their behaviour and not keep repeating old patterns.
- Help clients to *draw on their inner strengths and resources*, so that they can live their lives in harmony with their complex and rich inner world.

2   The Therapeutic Relationship in Cognitive Psychodynamic Therapy

In terms of the therapeutic relationship, we discussed in Chapter 3 how people strive to meet their attachment needs and develop human connection. However, many people feel insecure in their relationships. At the same time, many clients experience a pervasive sense of anxiety in their day-to-day lives. Going to meet a stranger to talk about intimate details of one's life in therapy is inherently anxiety provoking! Further, many clients have low self-esteem and perceive themselves to have low levels of personal efficacy. They may be defensive and expecting criticism. Therapists therefore need to be sensitive to these characteristics and develop a style which seeks to reassure and put people at ease. We need to word our interventions carefully, so that they are not wrongly construed, and seek to correct and reassure if they are. Rogers (1951) termed this attitude one of "unconditional positive regard", which conveys a non-judgemental stance. The therapist therefore models with the client a way of relating which is sensitive, non-defensive and non-judgemental.

As we discussed in Chapter 4, the way we relate to other people is based on our past experiences over many years. For most of us, our early childhood relationships will be critical. According to an example we used previously, if we experienced a harsh critical parent, this will have impacted on our sense of our self, but it will also impact on how we interact with others. If we perceive someone as being critical, this might arouse feelings of discomfort. We may routinely avoid people we perceive as critical. If we do have to interact with such people, we might adopt a strong, combative style. This is the notion of transference, where clients react to therapists not based on the current relationship but based on past relationships. As therapists, there is always the possibility we may experience something similar, where a client triggers a response in us, referred to as *countertransference*. Clients (and therapists) will differ in the extent to which their current interactions are coloured and affected by their past experiences. For many clients, their interactions with a therapist may be driven largely in that moment, with little influence from the past, and likewise for therapists. The relationship at that moment could be said to be real and genuine. For other clients, the interaction with the therapist may be strongly driven by triggers and past experience. In this case, the therapist can work with this aspect of the therapeutic experience, to help the client gain insight. As noted above, this would need to be done carefully, sensitively and non-judgementally. It can often be helpful to draw parallels with client experience outside of the therapy room.

Therefore, the therapist, in the therapeutic relationship, is modelling for the client a way of relating which is sensitive, non-defensive and real in that moment. This implies that the therapist will have done sufficient personal development work and therapy themselves so that they are aware of how their formative experiences have influenced the ways in which they behave in relationship. They will have personal insight into what the triggers are which might activate past learning and schemas. They will need to review this over the course of their work, as it is always possible that a new client will trigger some aspect of our former experience in a new way or which has not been previously activated. This may then prompt additional development/personal therapeutic work.

3   The Therapeutic Process

Most counselling and psychotherapy approaches tend to breakdown the process into three distinct phases. These are the assessment phase, the ongoing therapeutic working phase and the ending phase. These would also apply to a cognitive psychodynamic approach as described below.

3.1   Beginnings and Assessment

Most therapists will begin their initial sessions with a new client by going over the contractual details, discussing confidentiality issues and exploring the client's expectations. It can often be useful to ask if they have previous experience of therapy, as this can often drive their expectations. It can also be a useful pointer as to how the client might react to a particular approach. In cognitive psychodynamic terms, the client's previous experience of therapy might have been negative or positive, and this might then influence how they react to this particular episode of therapy.

We would recommend that therapists carry out a thorough and rigorous assessment, e.g. using a comprehensive approach such as that outlined by Ingram (2011). Ingram adopts the anagram BASIC SID (adapted from Lazarus's [1981] version) to remind therapists of the areas they might cover, where these stand for behaviour, affect, sensation, imagery, cognition, spirituality, interpersonal and drugs/biology. This is a useful framework for scoping out client issues. It reminds us, for example, that the chronic fatigue and lack of energy which many clients complain of can have a biological as well as a psychological origin.

Many therapists will ask at some point during an assessment "so what is it that brings you here today", giving the client the space to put in words what has brought them to the therapy room. In cognitive psychodynamic terms, this is giving the client the space to put into words their feelings of incongruence and inconsistency. It can often be useful to help clients bring these issues into focus by asking them what they hope to get out of the therapeutic work, and if they have specific goals in mind. Where client concerns are tied to very specific issues, they may state this very clearly. For example, a client that is trying to change a serious gambling habit might say they want to be able to go through life without spending large amounts of their money on gambling. They may be able to give quite specific goals, e.g. "be able to walk down the high street without feeling the urge to go into a betting shop". However, other clients may struggle to be as specific and may not be able to formulate any clear goals. Often clients in these circumstances will state their hopes in terms of symptoms or feelings, such as "I want to be able to go through life without feeling constantly anxious" or "I want life to have some meaning and sparkle again". For these clients, the incongruence and inconsistency are often deep-rooted, involving schemas and learning acquired over many years, leading to repetition of unhelpful patterns, often outside of client awareness.

From a cognitive psychodynamic perspective, the assessment therefore should lead to an initial understanding of the incongruence and inconsistency the client is feeling. As we illustrate in Fig. 1, this account is likely to be in terms of the way in which these become manifest in conscious cognitive thought processes, and the ways these are driven by the representational system, often implicitly. This then leads to various behavioural patterns, within which the tendencies of approach and avoidance will be evident.

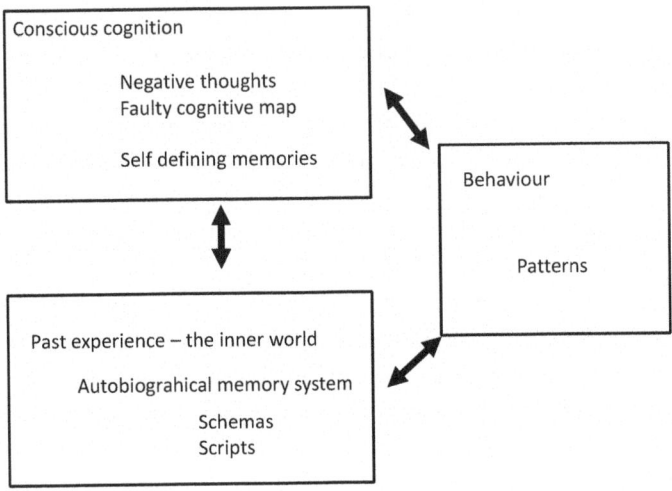

Fig. 1 The complex interplay of cognitive psychodynamic forces

From this initial formulation of the client's incongruence/inconsistency, a therapeutic plan can be put forward and negotiated with the client.[1]

– Where there are clear specific goals which lend themselves to *evidence-based strategies*, these might be put forward to the client. For example, specific anxieties are often helped significantly through cognitive behavioural techniques, and there is evidence that this can be more effective than other approaches (Wamplold, 2013). Having said that, in our experience people with specific anxieties will often benefit from looking back at their life course, and reviewing key events, which may have had an important impact on their adult coping strategies and ways of responding to anxiety and stress.[2]

---

[1]In Chapters 6–8, more details will be given on the assessment of the inner world in depressive disorders, traumatic disorders and anxiety disorders from the perspective of cognitive psychodynamics (see Tables 1 in Chapter 6, 2 in Chapter 7, and 2 in Chapter 8).

[2]See Chapter 8 on anxiety disorders.

- Where the incongruence is more diffuse and rooted in experience over many years, the therapeutic strategy may revolve around *exploring the inner world and past experiences*, reflecting on early environments and relationships, and working to understand how these have impacted on current experience, behaviour and relationships. The rationale here is to help clients gain insight and enable them to then adopt strategies which help them to break free from unhelpful patterns.

Hilary's assessment.
As mentioned in the initial summary, Hilary's presenting concern was that there was something unsatisfactory about her day to day relationships. She often felt that her interactions with friends and relatives left her feeling unhappy and was confused about why this was. So, for example Hilary would say:

> *Hilary: I don't know, it just seems to happen time and again. I get pulled into conversations, and I'm left feeling really confused at the end. I just don't really get what's going on.*
> *Therapist: Hm hmm, it feels like a pattern, it happens over and over, and at the end your confused, it's like not any particular feeling, just confusion, as if to say "how did that happen again?!"*
> *Hilary: yerr, like that, and I really want to know why it happens, so I can stop it happening again.*

As with many client's, Hilary was unable to be very specific about these issues, simply stating that she wanted her relationships to work out better, and for her to be happier as a result. It was agreed therefore that the initial approach to therapy would be to continue to explore Hilary's experiences in relationship, with a view to gaining insight into what was going on and how she could progress.

3.2 Ongoing Therapeutic Working

At the end of the initial assessment sessions, it should be clearer what the issues are that have brought the client to therapy/counselling. Where there are clear and specific issues, e.g. around the client experiencing disabling levels of anxiety in a particular situation, then it is likely that the approach to therapeutic working negotiated will reflect this. Specific strategies may be adopted such as use of relaxation prior to exposure to the anxiety-provoking situations. In other cases, where the issues are more diffuse, the approach may involve continued exploration, so that past patterns can be reflected on and related to current issues and ongoing concerns.

As the process of therapy unfolds, the client's hopes and goals for therapy may change. Clients with very specific goals focused on discrete problems may change as they progress and achieve their initial milestones. For example, a client with a fear of travelling by car following an accident may achieve their initial goal of being able to sit in a car as a passenger whilst it moves slowly around a car park. They might then wish to move onto a next step, such as being able to sit in the car whilst it moves at normal speed down a stretch of quiet road. Someone with more diffuse goals might come to refine these as they gain in insight and patterns become more evident. For example, someone with depression might say they want to be happier. As therapy progresses, they may reflect that some of their unhappiness relates to their avoidance of social contacts, and that this is due to their own feelings of lack of self-worth. They might then move on to reflect further on their feelings of self-worth. This could well focus on aspects of their early environment and messages they were given by their parents or guardians. They might move on to consider how they can enhance their self-esteem and at the same time look to increase their social contacts.

Ongoing Working with Hilary.
The sessions with Hilary focussed on her current relationships, to try and gain insight into the pattern which she was describing. Consistent with cognitive psychodynamic principles, there was also exploration of Hilary's past experience, to try and discern how her past learning and relationships may have led to the current dynamics evident in her current relations.

One particular aspect of Hilary's past experience seemed to be very relevant, as she describes below.

> *Hilary: I remember mum and dad were always very calm when they were together. There was never a raised voice in our house. You knew if you had done something wrong, and we'd get sent to our rooms, but there was never a raised voice. The divorce must have been one of the most friendly ever!*

Therapist: hmmm, so it's as if there was this expectation of peace and calm around, and never any raised voices? Not even with each other, when they were splitting up?

Hilary: yeh, I never knew them to shout or even raise their voices with each other - and I think that was the problem I had with mother after they split.

Therapist: even after, your mother still kept up this calm appearance? And that was difficult?

Hilary: yeah, because even when she brought a boyfriend round and he slapped me really hard for staying out and answering him back, she wouldn't get annoyed, or stick up for me.

Therapist: that sounds really difficult, as if your mum wasn't on your side and had put you in this situation?

Hilary: yeah, she never seemed to get it. I brought this up a few years later after they had split up and said how upset I had been about that incident - and she finally seemed to take it on board and got rid of the coat he had bought her, after I said it constantly reminded me of him.

The interesting point about this anecdote from Hilary is how she has been raised by parents who seemed to be very intolerant of strongly expressed emotions, and how raised voices were not allowed. Other anecdotes suggested that her parents avoided confrontation at all costs, and this seems to have then played a role in Hilary's mother's reaction when her boyfriend was excessive towards her daughter in his physical reaction over a discipline issue. This need for calm and avoidance of negative sensations seems to have played out in other ways for Hilary too as in the following excerpt:

Hilary: I can't tolerate bad things happening, sometimes I have to work really hard to find a way to turn things round, and it just uses up all my energy.

Therapist: ah ahh, so if something bad happens, you have to find a way to change it, make it positive?

Hilary: yeh, so a few months ago, I dropped my phone on the way to work, so the screen smashed, and it was basically unusable. I kept thinking about it all day, and how useless I was to have dropped it. The next day, I managed to get out in the lunch break and go round to the phone shop near the office. Because I'm on a contract, I had to pay for another phone, but they had just got a new model in and it was quite a bit cheaper than I thought it would be. So then I felt better, because I had a new phone, and it was way better than the one I dropped.

Therapist: ah ahh, so it's as though you find it really difficult to sit with a negative, you have to find a way to turn that around in your mind to a positive, like you might have dropped your phone, but so what you now have a new one, and its way better than the old one.

Hilary: exactly, and I have to do that all the time.

So we can see that Hillary finds negative sensations difficult, and that she has been brought up in an environment where expressing strong negative emotions is frowned upon. This then seems to play out in her day to relationships. Consider for example one interaction which has occurred between sessions:

Hilary: so I had another occasion this week where I was left feeling really awkward after talking to someone. After my phone broke last week, there were a few days where I wasn't able to text anyone, till I got my phone replaced. A friend texted me asking if we could meet up urgent as she had just had a big falling out with her boyfriend. Well, I never saw the text, so a few days later I saw her in town and she's like "oh don't speak to me, your never there when I need you, but if you need something I'm expected to come running". I'm like, ohh, yeah, but my phone broke, I never got your message" and she's like "oh yeah, always some excuse" and walked off. And I'm left feeling...... what?....

Therapist: OK, so it sounds like your friend is being really unreasonable there, and your left feeling quite confused, and not sure how that came about?

Hilary: yeah exactly, and it happens like that so often.

Therapist: hm hmm, and I wonder how you are left feeling at that point?

It soon became evident from looking at situations like this that Hillary's "confusion" was her way of labelling difficult emotions and not acting on them. With a little prompting it emerged that in fact one of her underlying feelings was one anger and being enraged at being so unfairly treated, and that this was an impulse she would never act upon.

In the following weeks, Hilary came to be much more aware of her negative feelings, and tentatively started to act upon these, by becoming more assertive. For example, she told her friend the next time they met that she had felt very unfairly treated, and that in fact their friendship was far less one sided than her friend had tried to suggest.

3.3   Ending

We do not see cognitive psychodynamic therapy as an approach which is open ended and likely to last for years, but at the same time we recognize that different clients have different degrees of need. Therefore, clients are likely to find therapy useful for differing lengths of time, and ideally therapists need to be flexible in relation to individuals. We also recognize, consistent with what we have outlined above, that client's views of their issues and goals will change as therapy progresses. It is therefore difficult to be precise with clients at the outset as to how long therapy will last, other than to say that different clients find that different numbers of sessions are enough, and this will be something that therapist and client will review as therapy progresses.

At some point, most clients will come to a view that they have explored their current issues to a depth which has led to a degree of resolution and insight which is sufficient at that point. This may also involve a judgement that further change in a particular issue is likely to be difficult or slow, and therefore a decision is made to park that issue for the time being. A satisfactory planned ending will therefore involve a discussion between the therapist and client about the progress being made, the extent to which goals and expectations have been met, and whether therefore this is an appropriate time to bring sessions to a close. This is not to say that the client may not choose to seek additional sessions at some point in the future, but that they feel comfortable with where they are at for the moment.

Therapists will have different approaches to ending with their clients. In our view, it is useful to review the course of therapy and the progress made, highlighting the various insights which have been gained. This then clarifies for the client the gains they have made from the cognitive psychodynamic way of working. We think it is also important to spend time looking to the future, considering how the client can use the insights they have gained to continue moving in the desired direction, and avoid falling back into unhelpful and counterproductive patterns.

For many client issues, it is important to consider the issue of relapse and how to look out for this and cope with it if necessary. In many problematic areas, e.g. substance use or gambling, relapse can be a very real risk, and not thinking about this in advance can lead to catastrophic failure if it should happen. Looking out for it and having a plan can make all the difference.

3.3.1 Ending with Hilary

Hilary was very open to the work she did in therapy and responded quickly to the insights gained. She was very receptive to the point that her upbringing had conditioned her to avoid negative sensations, and not to use a raised voice or get into conflict. She tentatively began to allow her sensations of anger and become more assertive in her interactions. The client ended after twelve sessions, suggesting that the insights gained were likely to helpful, and reduce her sense of confusion around everyday interactions.

4   Specific Client Issues

In this chapter, we have thought in general terms about the principles which guide cognitive psychodynamic therapy. These have been developed from our current knowledge of cognition, neuroscience, client issues and the wisdom gained from over one hundred years of people thinking about how to conduct psychotherapy. In the preceding chapters, we have touched on a number of specific client issues. For instance, in Chapter 2 we briefly addressed the neuroscience of depression and anxiety. In the following chapters, we will now look in detail at specific common presenting concerns by successively considering depression, anxiety and trauma. In each case, we will cover in more detail what a cognitive psychodynamic approach to this problem area might look like. We will look at both the theory, as well as the specifics of working therapeutically.

5   Concluding Remarks

Cognitive psychodynamic therapy combines theoretical principles from cognitive science and neuroscience with the clinical insights stemming from over one hundred years of the psychodynamic tradition. It recognizes that a significant number of issues which clients bring to psychotherapy are rooted in their experience and learning. The starting point is always the client's expression of their incongruence or feelings of inconsistency. This can sometimes lend itself to quite specific desired outcomes and goals. However, it is often the case that clients are not able to shape their psychological distress into clear goals. This reflects the situation where clients have learned unhelpful patterns of behaviour or ways of relating from their past. Allowing the client to explore their inner worlds and narratives, in the context of a supportive therapeutic relationship, will often lead to insights into these patterns. This in turn empowers the client to change these tendencies, and to develop new ways of responding.

The cognitive psychodynamic paradigm we have described is based on a comprehensive knowledge base drawn from contemporary psychology and neuroscience. This offers a holistic view of what it is to be human, as well as the phenomena of humans in relationship with each other. This theoretical base allows for the elaboration of what effective therapy should consist of. Our expectation is that it will be a rich tapestry for guiding and directing future research.

Points to Ponder

- It could be argued that the example given in this chapter around Hilary illustrates the important role which emotion plays in our everyday lives and relationships. Have you worked with clients where part of the issue being faced was around their processing of emotions? How did this play out in their case?
- No diagnostic label was given here for Hilary. If she had expressed her disquiet in a setting where labels are employed, what sort of labels might have been used?

- This chapter has set out the principles for cognitive psychodynamic therapy. To what extent are these consistent with your pre-existing thoughts about therapy or your established ways of working?
- What would you say might be the difficulties with, or gaps in, a cognitive psychodynamic way of working?

References

Cooper, M. (2019). *Integrating counselling and psychotherapy: Directionality, synergy and social change*. London, Thousand Oaks, New Delhi, and Singapore: Sage.

Ingram, B. L. (2011). *Clinical case formulations: Matching the integrative treatment plan to the client*. New York: Wiley.

Lapworth, P., & Sills, C. (2010). *Integration in counselling and psychotherapy* (2nd ed.). London, Thousand Oaks, New Delhi, and Singapore: Sage.

Lazarus, A. A. (1981). *The practice of multimodal therapy: Systematic, comprehensive, and effective psychotherapy*. New York: McGraw-Hill.

Rogers, C. R. (1951). *Client centred therapy*. London: Constable.

Wampold, B. E. (2013). *The great psychotherapy debate: Models, methods, and findings*. London: Routledge.

6

When Life Loses Its Lustre

1   Background

Many clients that seek counselling or psychotherapy will say in their initial session that they have been feeling low, and that this has been the case for some considerable time. In some cases, they will have already visited their medical practitioner, who may have offered to prescribe antidepressants. In other cases, this may not be the first time they have felt this way. They may have had similar episodes of feeling very low and may have previously sought help from therapists.

A diagnosis of depression is based on two main features. First is the experience of low mood over a prolonged period of time. Second is the loss of interest or pleasure in usual activities. These are the two key criteria, though a formal diagnosis does require additional symptoms (American Psychiatric Association, 2013). Deciding on whether someone meets these criteria often involves the use of symptom questionnaires such as the Patient Health Questionnaire (PHQ9)—Kroenke,

© The Author(s) 2019
T. Ward and A. Plagnol, *Cognitive Psychodynamics as an Integrative Framework in Counselling Psychology and Psychotherapy*,
https://doi.org/10.1007/978-3-030-25823-8_6

Spitzer, and Williams (2001)—or the Beck Depression Inventory (e.g. see Beck, Steer, & Brown, 1996, who compare the original and more recent versions). Thus, clinical depression involves an overwhelming loss of hope and low mood, plus loss of interest and pleasure in one's day-to-day concerns. This tells us something about the experience of being depressed, but it does not tell us about how people come to feel this way.

As Paykel (2008) outlines, there is a long-established view that depression can be divided into two main types. One, endogenous depression, seems to bear little relationship to what is going on in the person's life, whereas reactive depression can be seen as a response to adverse events or trauma. Paykel also discusses the association of the former with other complex presentations, e.g. schizoaffective disorder where there may be delusional beliefs or hallucinations. Reality seems to be more complex than this long-standing account would indicate. Brown, Harris, and Hepworth (1994) suggested for example that life history does not always allow for such a straightforward categorization. There does seem to be some evidence that early adverse life events could be linked to later development of depression (Heim, Owens, Plotsky, & Nemeroff, 1997), and the risk of being impacted by such events could be heightened by a genetic predisposition (Alexander et al., 2009). Genetic risk such as reported in the latter study is based on genes which are linked to the production of serotonin in the brain, which is the neurotransmitter targeted by most current antidepressants (e.g. see Wade, Lemming, & Hedegaard, 2002, for a typical clinical trial of a selective serotonin reuptake inhibitor [SSRI]). A cognitive view of this differential susceptibility which some people may have towards becoming depressed is that for some reason, perhaps linked to past events or life history, some people have a cognitive vulnerability, which makes them more susceptible to future stress (Lau, Segal, & Williams, 2004).

In the following sections, we will look in more detail at the range of factors which have been linked to depression, in terms of the forces which act upon people, and how these forces come to shape their inner world and thought processes.

2   Mapping the Contours of a Bleak Inner World

Cognitive reactivity is the tendency, when exposed to negative events, to activate negative internal memory states and schemas. The stronger this tendency in an individual, the greater the risk for multiple episodes of depression (Elgersma et al., 2015). According to the differential activation hypothesis (Lau, Segal, & Williams, 2004), negative childhood experiences may lead to negative information processing biases, resulting in the negative cognitive triad of thoughts about the self, future and the world (Beck & Alford, 2009). Later, stress will then lead to depression, dependent on the degree of activation and content of the negative representations. The risk of depression will depend upon the averseness of the stress, how uncontrollable it is perceived to be and whether this is then linked to global negative judgements about the self. According to these authors, once depression has been triggered, this then leads to further negative consequences such as increased structure and strength of negative beliefs and attitudes. There is evidence of a change in outlook occurring as a result of an episode of depression (Laidlaw & Davidson, 2001).

The hypothetical structure said to result from negative childhood experiences and lead to future processing biases is the negative schema (e.g. Gotlib, Krasnoperova, Yue, & Joormann, 2004 showed that people with depression show an attentional bias towards sad faces) and more particularly negative *self*-schemas. Segal (1988) gives a detailed outline of the self-schema concept in depression and reviews evidence for and against this account. Evidence supporting this view in terms of development includes Kelvin, Goodyer, Teasdale, and Brechin (1999), who showed that adolescents high in emotionality, subject to negative mood induction, elicited greater numbers of negative self-descriptors. Friedmann, Lumley, and Lerman (2016) showed that adolescents with negative self-schemas when first assessed had a tendency to be more depressed when assessed again some time later (note that schemas here are referring to Young, Klosko, & Weishaar [2003] notion of maladaptive schemas). In terms of connections to depression, Disner, Shumake, and Beevers (2017) showed that more negative self-schemas were associated with increased depression. They hypothesized this was due to increased attentional bias, leading to depression getting worse over time. In terms of the progression of depression, Dozois and Dobson (2003) found that where people had experienced more episodes of depression, this was linked to increasingly structured negative material and less connected positive material. A later study (Seeds & Dozois, 2010) suggested that the increasing organization of negative material led to a greater negative reaction to adverse life events. Thus, these studies illustrate the point being made above, that episodes of depression lead to further structural changes, in a sort of negative feedback loop.

Studies focusing on self-schemas have used many and varied methodologies. The recent popularity of techniques designed to elicit implicit processes has led to this methodology being applied in this field also. Franck, De Raedt, and De Houwer (2008) replicated several previous studies, in failing to find any significant differences between people with depression and controls on an implicit association test. Such tasks examine people's reaction times to infer how strongly they associate concepts such as "sad" with self-reference terms such as "me". A more recent study by Dentale et al. (2016) did however find impressive correlations between the Depression Implicit Association Test (DIAT) and validation measures such as the Beck Depression Inventory. The positive results in this case may have been due to the highly heterogeneous sample, i.e. people with depression and university students, thus increasing the variance in the data.

A possible criticism of this body of work on self-schemas is that the construct is rather narrow. It almost certainly neglects the many and varied ways in which people's past experiences become encoded into their inner worlds in such a way as to influence their future perceptions and experiences. For example, as noted by Segal (1988), past relationships are likely to be very important. Interestingly, Blatt and Zuroff (1992) noted that interpersonal issues were likely to be an important second dimension underlying depression, alongside negative self-concepts. As we noted in the chapter on memory and schemas, the representational system could include many aspects of experience, including typical parental coping strategies, expectations and rules about living, prohibitions on proscribed ways of being, etc. All of this will be enmeshed in a unique constellation, specific to an individual client.

These implicit representation structures will shape and influence the conscious contents which surface within the theatre of the mind (Baars, 1997). These conscious contents will often consist of autobiographical memories. As we saw in Chapter 4, the neural basis of the autobiographical memory system is being mapped out (Svoboda, McKinnon, & Levine, 2006). Interestingly, this neural system may be responsible for a number of cognitive processes linked to theatre of the mind operations, including internal focusing (Spreng, Mar, & Kim, 2009).

Evidence shows that people with depression will experience a number of effects in relation to their autobiographical memories. For example, they tend to recall fewer positive memories, and their memories tend to be less specific (Lemogne et al., 2009; Williams & Broadbent, 1986; Williams & Scott, 1988). They also recall more negative memories (Lemogne et al., 2006). Kuyken and Brewin (1995) found that autobiographical memory tended to be over general in people with depression where there was a history of abuse.

These observed effects in autobiographical memory could be due to a number of processes. The negative self-representations found in implicit memory could produce processing biases, such that negative events tend to become a focus of attention. Another possibility is that active elements of the negative self-representations could prime negative memories through association. In terms of the lack of specifics and over-generalization, this could be a defence mechanism, to avoid focusing on painful specific memories, thus memory retrieval could be prevented from reaching down to discrete incidents (poor recall strategy was one suggestion put forward by Williams and Broadbent [1986] to account for their results whilst Whalley, Rugg, and Brewin [2012] suggested susceptibility to distractors).

Given these effects in autobiographical memory, several studies have suggested possible intervention strategies targeted at this aspect of the condition. Williams, Teasdale, Segal, and Soulsby (2000) suggested that mindfulness training helped clients to notice their memories non-judgementally, and thus, they would be less likely to abandon search strategies. Hitchcock, Werner-Seidler, Blackwell, and Dalgleish

(2017) reviewed an array of studies which used various memory training strategies. These included practice in accessing positive memories and rehearsal of thinking about future possible positive scenarios. Their overall conclusion was that the evidence supports memory training as a useful strategy for people with depression.

So far, we have seen that in many people with depression, there is evidence of an inner world characterized by negative representations of the self. Stressful life events can activate these structures, leading to depression, which in turn leads to the inner world becoming even more negatively structured. This impacts on people's perceptions of the world, as well as their recall of past events. It seems that to avoid painful memories, people's recall of their past becomes more general and less specific, as if they are avoiding recall of particular events (probably very much the case in the case of Kuyken and Brewin's [1995] participants who had suffered actual abuse). Thus, the inner world becomes more and more restricted, with less and less focus on detail. The processing bias results in memory recall being negative, and the loss of specifics means that positive memories become cut off. As we will now see below, similar tendencies can play out in the client's life, leading to increasing restriction of activities.

3   Approach/Avoidance and Behavioural Activation

An early theory of depression suggested that if subjected to repeated adverse circumstances, people would become despondent and cease responding to their environment (Seligman, 1972). In Chapter 3, we saw how behavioural responses could be broadly seen as approach or avoidance oriented. These correspond to the behavioural inhibition and behavioural activation systems outlined by Jorm et al. (1998). Pinto-Meza et al. (2006) found that in depressed participants, the behavioural inhibition system was more active than in controls, whilst the behavioural activation system was less active. The latter was also found in people recovering from depression, suggesting that behavioural activation may generally be reduced in people susceptible to depression. The implications of this are that people with depression will be more sensitive to, and avoidant of, experiences they anticipate being unpleasant. At the same time, they will be less inclined to seek out positive experiences. This is a similar parallel to the position outlined above in relation to memory, where people may avoid certain types of memory in expectation of painful consequences, but thus also depriving themselves of positive experiences.

Behavioural activation is an approach which involves working with clients to structure and schedule positive activities into their lives (Santos et al., 2017). It is widely used with people who have mild to moderate depression (Chartier & Provencher, 2013). It has also been found to be as effective as medication and more effective than cognitive therapy, in people with severe depression (Dimidjian, Barrera, Martell, Munoz, & Lewinsohn, 2011). For many clients, the gains can be sudden and dramatic. For example, Masterson et al. (2014) found that over 40% of their sample showed sudden gains, often within a short number of sessions. These clients tended to have better overall outcomes. The authors suggested that this might reflect increased goal-driven activity and self-activation (as opposed to relying on therapist direction).

There is good evidence in favour of helping clients to increase their levels of engagement and thus overcome their decreased behavioural activation. This enables them to benefit from positive reinforcement and is very worthwhile. In effect, this is an active strategy for helping people to start re-shaping the contours of their inner world and providing them with a catalogue of positive experiences which can be activated to overcome any negative bias. As they increase their repertoire and range of engagement with the world, their self-schema becomes less negative and their sense of self-worth increases. The inner world becomes less dark and less foreboding.

4   Pointers from the Psychotherapy Literature

We have seen from the section above on behavioural activation that helping people to structure positive experiences and activities can be helpful for people with depression. What other approaches have been shown to be effective? In thinking about this question, it is often helpful to look at meta-analyses. These are studies which collate lots of clinical research studies together, allowing them to aggregate data and compare different approaches. There are a number of recently published meta-analyses in relation to psychotherapeutic approaches to depression.

Given the emphasis in the literature on negative self-schemas and biases in cognitive processing, it would be surprising if cognitive behaviour therapy was not found to be effective. In fact, there is now probably more evidence in favour of this approach than any other (e.g. Tolin, 2010). Note here that we are simply reflecting the volume of research which exists on this approach, not necessarily implying it is superior to other approaches.

A perspective which is often contrasted with cognitive behaviour therapy is psychodynamic therapy. Typically, this involves the therapist helping the client to think about unresolved conflicts linked to past relationships. Leichsenring (2001) found psychodynamic approaches to be as effective as cognitive behaviour therapy, although the number of studies they were able to find was small. Driessen et al. (2010) found rather more studies, with twenty-three in their analysis. They found psychodynamic approaches to be effective, with large effect sizes. Whilst they noted that other therapies were often better in terms of immediate post-treatment effects, all were equivalent at follow up. Fonagy et al. (2015) looked at long-term psychoanalytic approaches to treatment-resistant depression. Whilst this did not produce benefits over control conditions at the end of treatment, there were longer term benefits on follow up. Thus, there seems to be a view across several studies that psychodynamic approaches appear to produce longer lasting effects, which seems to be worthy of further research and follow up.

There have been several large meta-analyses in recent years comparing multiple therapeutic approaches. Cuijpers, van Straten, Andersson, and van Oppen (2008) looked at interpersonal therapy, behavioural activation, cognitive behaviour therapy, problem-solving, social skills training, psychodynamic therapy and supportive counselling. They found all to be effective and generally equivalent except that interpersonal was slightly better, and the dropout rate in cognitive behaviour therapy was greater. A similar study by Cuijpers et al. (2011) focused on interpersonal therapy, finding it to be significantly better than control conditions, but no different to other approaches in overall efficacy. Finally, Barth et al. (2016) conducted a large network meta-analysis (a complex statistical technique which allows inference across studies), comparing the same seven therapies looked at by Cuijpers et al. (2008). They also concluded that all seven therapies produced significant effects compared to control, with effect sizes ranging from moderate to large. They concluded that given the larger amount of data available, these effects were most robust for cognitive behaviour therapy, interpersonal therapy and problem-solving.

The overall conclusion seems to be that all therapeutic approaches to depression are potentially useful. The evidence for a traditional psychodynamic stance is slightly weaker, though this clearly benefits some and may produce long-lasting effects. The interpersonal approach also seems to be well supported. This fits with Blatt and Zuroff's (1992) suggestion that depression often arises from two sources, negative self-characterization and interpersonal issues.

5 A Cognitive-Psychodynamic Approach to Depression

As we outlined at the beginning of this chapter, depression tends to be characterized by a general loss of hope, pervasive lowering of mood and a failure to derive reward and pleasure from everyday activities. These characteristics are reflected in common rating scales of depression such as the Beck Depression Inventory. In such measures, clients are invited to indicate if they agree or disagree that statements such as "I feel tearful all the time" are true of them. However, the individual histories of clients which bring them to this point are many and varied, with each person having their own unique constellation of previous life experiences.

As we saw in Chapter 2, emotion plays a significant role in our everyday cognitive processing and decision-making. We use our anticipated emotional responses to guide our actions. At the same time, as we saw in Chapter 3, frustration in reaching our goals and meeting our basic psychological needs will lead to psychological tension. A similar state will be evoked by lack of consistency and congruence in our inner world.

Thus, clients with depression are likely to have experienced frustration in meeting their basic psychological needs over a considerable period of time, often since childhood. These difficulties may well trigger negative memory structures around self, acquired during development or resulting from previous trauma. Their *low mood* and lack of enjoyment may have caused them to restrict their activities, and this can also be reflected by a lack of internal engagement with specific memories.

To highlight the full value of a cognitive psychodynamic framework, by integrating the contributions of the approaches we have mentioned—behavioural activation, cognitive psychotherapy, psychodynamic approach, interpersonal therapy—let's go a little deeper to understand the inner world of a depressed client.

Mood can be understood as the basic emotional tone that reflects the degree of congruence/consistency of the active part of the inner world (Plagnol, 2002, 2004). An incongruence between active fragments of the inner world generates an internal tension,[1] notably when there is a conflict between a misfortune (e.g. a break-up with a deeply loved partner) and the memories of happiness. If the tension is too high, defence processes are triggered, removing too painful representations from consciousness (more exactly, from the "theatre of the mind" or "window of presence"[2]). Such defence processes provide protection against pain, but leave active fragments of representation in memory, which are not harmoniously integrated into the inner world and make the subject vulnerable. Such a vulnerability is aggravated:

- if the misfortune strikes the heart of the inner world, the client's history has forged it (e.g. the departure of the spouse/husband and children after years of living together);
- if the misfortune is anticipated as irreversible (e.g. the spouse/husband has made a new life with another), with no possible congruence on the horizon of the window of presence (in other words, loss of any hope of a peaceful life).

---

[1]In the next chapter on traumatic disorders, we will introduce a Principle of Unification (or Principle of Congruence/Consistency) according to which the representational system constantly tends to minimize the tension induced by mismatches within the inner active world.

[2]See Chapter 2.

In such conditions, the inner world is painfully closed both in the past and in the future, as is the case for the too famous "Unhappiest One" described by Kierkegaard (1843/1992). Every mental event is associated with a memory of what is lost and causes a wave of pain, all the more acute as there is no horizon for a solution. A natural defence is then a retraction of the inner world: as we have pointed out, there is an inhibition of mental processes in depression (and sometimes even a mental life freeze), with a global restriction of life in the outer world (behavioural inhibition). In the most severe cases, the inner world has become a "dark well" (a metaphor often used by depressed people). Indeed, a well offers protection against events, but at a terrible price—to the extreme, death by starvation—and if the subject tries to get out of it, reactivating what is lost triggers a wave of pain, therefore a relapse.

However, the despair of the subject often seems disproportionate to the unfortunate circumstances. Moreover, how can we explain the alteration in self-esteem that is perhaps the most striking feature of depression? As Freud (1917/1957) put it, the only possible explanation is a resonance of real circumstances with a more unconscious loss. Indeed, in any resistant depression, we can find the ancient loss of a founding ideal, associated with the basic organization of the inner world, for example a breakdown of the parental home.[3] Somewhere in the past, a flaw occurred in a "founding space" (typically dependent on parental figures), which was the key to a unified world and a basic sense of safety. As a rule, the roots of a resistant depression thus go back to an ancient split in the inner world to protect the ideal of the childhood home from misfortune, with a corresponding split of the Self between a bad Self (which took guilt on its shoulders, which gave an explanation for the misfortune[4]) and a heroic Self (which overcame the pain). Such an ancient situation of misfortune is at the origin of the development of negative schemas that later undermine the inner world of the adult, especially if losses in adolescence or in young adulthood have reinforced these schemas.

---

[3]As we will see in more detail in the next chapter, the ordinary inner world is often organized according to a fundamental intuition, the ideal of the Home, commonly associated with an ideal projection of the house where family happiness can unfold without clouds. (Remember Hilary's case in Chapter 5, her "expectation of peace and calm" at home, and the impact on her life of such an expectation even after the split of the parental home).

[4]Better an explanation than no explanation at all, which would mean an uncontrollable world. On the internalization of faults in a child, see Chapter 3, Sect. 6 and Sullivan (2013).

A psychodynamic-cognitive approach is therefore particularly interesting in resistant depression, to approach the inner world as a whole, as it has been shaped by a singular history. The therapist is attentive not only to the recent circumstances evoked by the subject, but also to the gaps in his or her explicit history,[5] which often outline the older roots of depression, and only become explicit during therapy, but which must be approached with caution during the therapy, once a solid therapeutic framework is established whilst respecting the subject's defences, to overcome a therapeutic blockage and the risk of relapse. For example, after a classic behavioural and cognitive approach has led to initial advances and the uncovering of pathogenic schemas, it is often necessary, in the case of persistent depressive vulnerability, to approach the subject's inner world and history in greater depth (Plagnol & Mirabel-Sarron, 2006). A dynamic cognitive perspective is then valuable in clarifying the extent of mental restructuring required to re-organize the inner world and recreate a coherent narrative of life with an open future.

6   Assessment

As outlined in Chapter 5, the starting point to working in a cognitive-psychodynamic way with a client who feels they are depressed would be to conduct one or more assessment sessions. This would involve a comprehensive overview of the client's concerns, typically using a framework such as that outlined by Ingram (2011). Clients will often refer to their low mood and often describe one or more negative

---

[5]It is frequent that from the first interview the client mentions painful distant situations, but no longer seems to attach importance to them as if they have been overcome. This was the case with M. C., a 26-year-old man, who was followed for several years for depressive episodes, although he was a very gifted, courageous and endearing person. Mr. C. had mentioned "in passing" during the first interview that his mother had been in a psychiatric hospital for a long time after his father had left home, but that fortunately his grandmother had affectionately cared for him: the collapse of the parental home was not a problem for him, he did not come to see a therapist for that. It was only after eighteen months of therapy that M. C.'s heroic Self was able to express the painful reality of his childhood, allowing therapeutic advances.

events which they may feel is related to this. On the other hand, some clients may not be able to describe any recent precipitating factors. It is possible that they will have previously visited their general practitioner and in some cases will have been prescribed antidepressants, which they may or may not still be taking. Failing to derive benefits from such medication is often what triggers clients to seek talking therapy. In our experience of working with clients with low mood, they may struggle to articulate specific goals. Not feeling low all the time and wanting to enjoy life again may well be the general way in which they express their hopes for the future.

We present in Table 1 some first steps towards exploring the inner world in depressive disorders from a cognitive-psychodynamic perspective, including for the therapist the importance of also considering his/her own inner world.

Table 1 First steps towards exploring the inner world in depressive disorders from the perspective of cognitive psychodynamics

First approach of the client's inner world
– Identify the spatial metaphors used by the client for family and professional life ("life course", "path", "home", etc.), disease ("no way out"), therapeutic encounter ("support", etc.);
– Take particular account of the metaphors involving light ("bleakness", "darkness", "pit", "wells", etc.), inhibition ("slowing down", "retraction", "cold", "freezing", etc.), fragility of the inner world ("cracks", "fractures", "split", etc.)
– What do these metaphors reflect about his/her active inner world? About his/her deeper inner world?
– Are there basic beliefs that underlie some of these metaphors?
– Is the client's inner world unified? Is there a keystone that gives meaning to life? How are self-schemas constructed?
– Are there any significant gaps in person's history? Potential traumatic events in the past?
– Is it possible to use some of the metaphors identified above with the client to make him/her aware of some essential features of his/her own inner world?
– What precautions should be taken?
– What are the links between the inner world and its environment («outer» world)?

(continued)

Table 1 (continued)

Circumstances of the depression, traumatic factors and effects on the inner world
– What are the triggering circumstances, however slight, for depressive symptoms?
– Are there ruminations about these circumstances? Active and painful memories? A hidden traumatic disorder (i.e. a re-experiencing syndrome still active)?
– How can you describe the incongruence between these circumstances/ruminations and the prior inner world?
– What are the subject's apprehensions (repetition of misfortunes? intractable pain? suffering until death?) What is the role of his/her imagination? Can he/she recognize it?
– How can the client describe the changes that the symptoms have produced in his or her inner world?
– Does the subject feel that basic beliefs have been disrupted?
– Does he/she still have a horizon? Does he/she think about dying?
– Are the circumstances sufficient to explain depressed mood and impaired self-esteem?
– What moves or blocking points are suggested his/her emotions?
– How does the subject feel about the therapeutic space between his/her inner world and the outer world? Is he/she in a safe place?

Resonances with the past
– Are there some detectable resonances between the triggering circumstances and past events?
– Does the subject spontaneously evoke older events? What time did they come back? Are they still active? What have been their effects on the inner world? What are the symbolic links with the current circumstances?
– What hypotheses can be made about the "roots" of the depressive vulnerability? Does the subject evoke these spontaneously?
– Are there some self-defining memories? Do they reflect the self-schemas?
– How to characterize the childhood home? The Ideal of the Self?
– How to characterize the parental figures in childhood? Protective or defective?
– Are there some signs of old cracks or flaws? Had there been real misfortunes? Or imagined? Has the childhood home been split?
– Was there any guilt felt? Did the child attribute the burden of a fault to himself/herself for explaining misfortunes? Were there any effects on self-esteem? Has he/she developed "heroic" attitudes? Did he/she seek recognition for that?
– What changes took place during adolescence and young adulthood (educational and vocational choices, romantic encounters, desire or not to leave the parental home, etc.)? Were there any difficult or even traumatic circumstances (disappointments, break-ups, interruption of studies, parental death, etc.)?
– What degree of fidelity does the subject feel for the parental home and the associated Ideal? Was he/she considering another home for himself/herself? Was there any obstacle before the triggering circumstances? Has it changed since that event?

(continued)

Table 1 (continued)

How is the therapist's inner world affected?
– What are the emotional sensations felt by the therapist?
(pity, feeling of helplessness, exhaustion, anger, boredom, etc.)
– How can the therapist's inner world reflect the client's inner world?
– What are the possible limits of empathy? (e.g. « dark areas », unspeakable
   painful bodily or mental experiences, gender or age or social gaps, etc.)

What objectives should be set for the reconfiguration of the inner world?
– Bring forward again some spatial metaphors: can the therapist glimpse
   "openings" of the inner worldinner world? What horizons can be proposed?
– How can these proposals be taken into account within the client's inner
   worldinner world?
– Will changes in basic beliefs be necessary?
– Can a unified world be found again? What are the specific obstacles to such
   unification?
– What are the subject's untapped resources? Is there any potential for
   post-depression growth?
– Are there accessible points of support such as social models or spiritual
   references?
– What precautions should be taken to create a solid therapeutic framework?
– What steps and timelines can be outlined for a recovery process?
– What would be the dangers of such a process?

At the end of the assessment period, it will most likely be evident
that low mood and loss of morale are the dominant client themes. There
may be evidence of negative thinking patterns, typically around the
self, world and future. The client may have withdrawn from the world
to some extent, both internally and externally. It may be the case that
they have developed a negative response bias. This may be evident in
a tendency to see the world in negative terms and to focus on negative
events. It may be apparent from talking of themselves that they have
a pervasive negative self-image, sometimes clearly rooted in childhood,
from the outset. This is not always obvious at earlier sessions, as clients
may compensate for this negative view of themselves, and they may
have striven in their lives for recognition

The offer to clients presenting with such a constellation of negative
mood and thinking will therefore be to explore his/her inner world
and reflect in more detail on their current life circumstances and

personal history, being careful to challenge negative thinking and out-look. Where clients have stopped approaching positive experiences and are avoiding situations they fear to be negative, active strategies can be encouraged to counter these. As discussed above (Dimidjian et al., 2011), the evidence suggests that re-engagement can have rapid and sig-nificant impacts on client mood. At the same time, clients are encour-aged to reflect on patterns of relationship and behavioural repertoires which might have a bearing on their current difficulties. The aim here is for clients to be able to increase insight where relevant, so that they can challenge negative thinking and work to build new patterns and response tendencies. In many cases, the aims and goals of therapy may change as sessions progress, as insight increases.

The assessment of Peter.
Peter was a middle-aged man who by his own account had been very successful in his career. He had started off in a company on the shop floor with no responsibilities, but over the years had gradually worked his way up and was now a regional sales director. He got married in his early twenties to a young lady that he worked with. He reported being very much in love at the outset, but wondered if they would have got married as quickly as they did if it had not been for his partner becoming pregnant. Over the years he felt that they had drifted apart, and in the later years he reported not being faithful on several occa-sions when away on business trips, though his partner never suspected this. Eventually they split up. At the time of the assessment, he had been divorced for seven years. In this time, he had been through sev-eral unsuccessful relationships. He was beginning to wonder if he would ever have another long-lasting relationship, and whether maybe there was something wrong with him. He felt quite lonely in the evenings and experienced intense sadness. A few years before he had approached his doctor who had prescribed antidepressants, but these did not seem to work. He therefore decided to come and try counselling. His stated goal was to try and find out what he was doing wrong and work out how to have a satisfying relationship again. At the time of the assessment, he had stopped trying to meet anyone, as he felt his attempts were likely to be unsuccessful.

In this example, we can see that Peter meets the classic definition of depression, in that he experiences low mood, and he no longer finds his day to day activities pleasurable. At one time he took great pride in his work, but this now seemed valueless as he had no one to share his ups and downs with. He also has negative views of himself, wondering if he is somehow to blame for a run of unsuccessful relationships, and this also carries into his view of the future, wondering if he will ever have a successful relationship again.

In classic cognitive terms, we can see that Peter has a negative worldview, which includes negative takes on himself and the future. His negative experiences have led him to start closing down his activities, not seeking to meet new people and expecting a negative outcome. On a positive note, Peter had not cut down on all social activities. He still met an old friend during the week to play squash, and cycled with a club at the weekends.

After the assessment, it was agreed that in further sessions Peter would explore his recent relationships and his reactions. At the same time, it was suggested that it might be useful to reflect on his earlier life, to see how previous patterns from his past might be playing out in his current interactions with people and potential partners.

In terms of the diagram we presented in chapter five, we can represent Peter's difficulties as follows (Fig. 1).

7   Ongoing Work with Clients

The initial sessions following the assessment period are likely to focus on exploring the client's day-to-day experience. This will often involve looking at their conscious cognitive thoughts and reflecting on how these link to their day-to-day activities. This can then lead to a consideration of the extent to which they are founded in reality and have a solid basis. The therapist role is often to challenge the validity of such negative thinking and allow the client to see how such thoughts may reflect a negative bias they have built up or negative views they hold about themselves.

As the work progresses, in many cases it will become evident that the negative world view and bias are long standing. This can lead to a

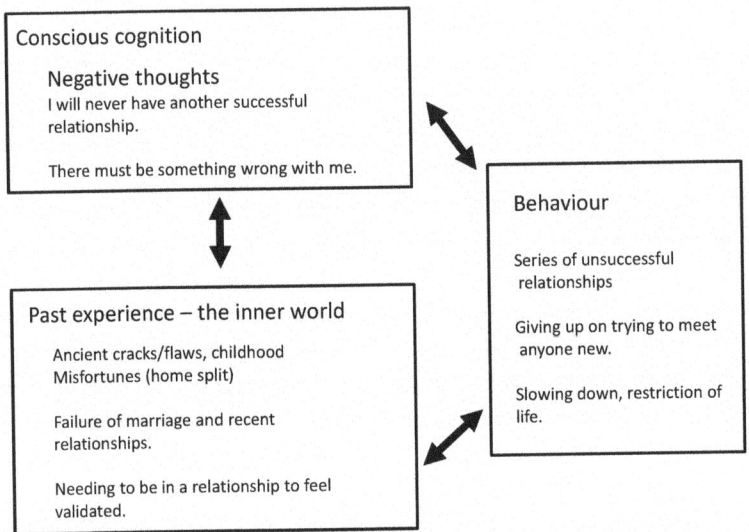

Fig. 1 Cognitive psychodynamic forces—the case of Peter

fruitful consideration of earlier experiences. Recollection of key self-defining memories (see Chapter 4) can be very revealing in giving an indication of the overall tone of people's early childhood environment. Where patterns and behavioural repertoires do become evident, clients can be encouraged to consider how these increased insights can be used to their advantage, so that they can build new patterns and ways of responding and avoid the old less helpful patterns.

Ongoing work with Peter.
The initial sessions with Peter further reinforced what had emerged during the assessment phase. He was demoralised, felt that he would never have another successful relationship, and that his future would therefore be lonely and unrewarding. At some level he felt that this was down to him, that somehow, he was doing something wrong. During the day at work, he could ward off these feelings. It was most acute in the evenings, when he came home and was by himself.

After several sessions, Peter began to talk more about his early experiences, and his relationships with his parents. Take this interaction for example:

Therapist: so your parents split up when you were about nine years old, and you and your younger sisters lived with your mother?

Peter: yeah that's right. Mum had a part time job, but it seemed we never had much money, we were always scrimping. It's really hard when you're the one at school that stands out, that never has the right kit they need.

Therapist: hm hmm, you really noticed how difficult it was.

Peter: yeah - and then mum met another bloke, who eventually became my step dad, but that didn't seem to change things much - he had a daughter of his own, so she was the one that got all the attention.

What this interaction and others illustrate is the key event in Peter's life of his parents splitting up. At the same time, both his maternal and paternal grandparents had been happily married for many years. These events seem to have been internalised by Peter in such a way that on the one hand he felt that people should always try to stay together where children were involved, and on the other that not being able to maintain a relationship was a personal failing.

The other striking aspect of Peter's story is the way in which his outward success is not matched by his internal self-representations, as shown here:

Peter: I remember we were away on holiday one time. We didn't have many holidays, but I think grandad must have paid for it. I used to really enjoy football, it was one of the few things I was good at - school was a bit of a washout for me. Anyway, there was a five a side football competition, and my side got through to the final. I scored most of the goals, including the final one of the match, and we got a cup. Mum said she would come and watch, but she never came near. She never even asked later how it had gone. I was gutted.

Therapist: hmm hmm, its as though she never showed you much attention.... You must have been left wondering if she was very proud of you?

Peter: exactly - I was the one that was no good at school, I was the one that no one expected to ever amount to anything.

From this interaction, we can see how Peter had a very low self-image and self-esteem. His successful career had allowed him to combat this to some extent, but his recent relationship difficulties seemed to be allowing this insecurity to come through in this aspect of his life.

8   Ending

Given that clients with depression often have long-standing and deeply rooted negative self-images and relational patterns, the therapeutic work can often take some time, and clients may not feel they have fully resolved their difficulties at the time they decide to end.

In our view, it is useful to review with clients in the ending session the journey they have been on. This will likely involve the negative thinking patterns which have been uncovered, and how these can be countered. It may involve reviewing the importance of engagement and maintaining positive and reinforcing activities. It will often involve reviewing the long-standing patterns and dispositions which the client has become aware of, and thinking about how to counter these, and not revert back to old patterns or fall into old traps.

Reviewing how to continue to maintain a positive outlook and disposition can often be important. In recent years, mindfulness has become widely used as an approach which can help people who have been depressed to maintain a more positive outlook and not relapse into depression. In our cognitive-psychodynamic model of the mind (see Chapter 2), the unconscious representational system contains negative self-schemas, which trigger negative automatic thoughts or conscious cognitions, in the theatre of the mind, or global workspace. These then lead to adverse changes in behaviour. Mindfulness trains people to simply observe this process and to disinvest these negative conscious cognitions of emotional energy. Thus, when they recur in future (as they are likely to given how ingrained and pervasive negative self-schemas are), the client has a chance through mindfulness of disengaging from them and not being drawn back into a spiral of negative thinking and reduced behavioural repertoire.

Ending with Peter.
In the final sessions with Peter, there was reflection on the negative thoughts he had initially expressed about himself and relationships. There was also some review of how this was linked to his early experiences, of his parents' divorce, family expectations around relationships, and his feeling that his mother did not value his achievements and tended to be relentlessly critical.

There was discussion of how he could move forwards and challenge his negative thinking should it recur. At that point, he had recently started to engage with dating again, and was in the early stages of a relationship. He was determined to take this slowly and felt that he had started to re-evaluate what he was looking for in a relationship. To an extent he wondered whether some of his partners in the past had embodied elements of his critical mother.

9   Concluding Remarks

Depression is characterized by low mood and for many clients reflects a substantial period of time where they have felt frustrated in meeting their basic psychological needs.

In many cases, the client's history suggests negative events or trauma in the past and a developmental environment, which resulted in feelings of negative self-worth. In later life, this can lead to expectation of negative outcomes and resignation.

Exploration of the client's inner world can shed light on this negative focus and allow them to build a more positive outlook and new more positive conceptions of themselves. This can be facilitated with behavioural activation strategies, helping clients to restructure their inner worlds through increased pleasurable activities and positive feedback.

Points to Ponder

- In your experience, have clients with low mood tended to have negative self-schemas?
- To what extent is re-engagement important? Is this something you have tended to do with clients? How would you help clients to structure this and if necessary find the motivation?
- Are people's early relationships always important in determining negative moods? Do the roots of negative self-schemas and relational schemas often go back to childhood with, for example, a split in the parental home?

References

Alexander, N., Kuepper, Y., Schmitz, A., Osinsky, R., Kozyra, E., & Hennig, J. (2009). Gene–environment interactions predict cortisol responses after acute stress: Implications for the etiology of depression. *Psychoneuroendocrinology, 34*(9), 1294–1303.

American Psychiatric Association. (2013). *Diagnostic and statistical manual of mental disorders (DSM-5®)*. Washington, DC: American Psychiatric Association.

Baars, B. J. (1997). In the theatre of consciousness: Global workspace theory, a rigorous scientific theory of consciousness. *Journal of Consciousness Studies, 4*(4), 292–309.

Barth, J., Munder, T., Gerger, H., Nüesch, E., Trelle, S., Znoj, H., ... & Cuijpers, P. (2016). Comparative efficacy of seven psychotherapeutic interventions for patients with depression: A network meta-analysis. *Focus, 14*(2), 229–243.

Beck, A. T., & Alford, B. A. (2009). *Depression: Causes and treatment*. Philadelphia: University of Pennsylvania Press.

Beck, A. T., Steer, R. A., & Brown, G. K. (1996). Beck depression inventory-II. *San Antonio, 78*(2), 490–498.

Blatt, S. J., & Zuroff, D. C. (1992). Interpersonal relatedness and self-definition: Two prototypes for depression. *Clinical Psychology Review, 12*(5), 527–562.

Brown, G. W., Harris, T. O., & Hepworth, C. (1994). Life events and endogenous depression: A puzzle reexamined. *Archives of General Psychiatry, 51*(7), 525–534.

Chartier, I. S., & Provencher, M. D. (2013). Behavioural activation for depression: Efficacy, effectiveness and dissemination. *Journal of Affective Disorders, 145*(3), 292–299.

Cuijpers, P., Geraedts, A. S., van Oppen, P., Andersson, G., Markowitz, J. C., & van Straten, A. (2011). Interpersonal psychotherapy for depression: A meta-analysis. *American Journal of Psychiatry, 168*(6), 581–592.

Cuijpers, P., van Straten, A., Andersson, G., & van Oppen, P. (2008). Psychotherapy for depression in adults: A meta-analysis of comparative outcome studies. *Journal of Consulting and Clinical Psychology, 76*(6), 909–923.

Dentale, F., Grano, C., Muzi, M., Pompili, M., Erbuto, D., & Violani, C. (2016). Measuring the automatic negative self-schema: New evidence for the construct and criterion validity of the Depression Implicit Association. *Self and Identity, 15*(5), 599–613.

Dimidjian, S., Barrera, M., Jr., Martell, C., Munoz, R. F., & Lewinsohn, P. M. (2011). The origins and current status of behavioral activation treatments for depression. *Annual Review of Clinical Psychology, 7,* 1–38.

Disner, S. G., Shumake, J. D., & Beevers, C. G. (2017). Self-referential schemas and attentional bias predict severity and naturalistic course of depression symptoms. *Cognition and Emotion, 31*(4), 632–644.

Dozois, D., & Dobson, K. (2003). Brief report: The structure of the self-schema in clinical depression: Differences related to episode recurrence. *Cognition and Emotion, 17*(6), 933–941.

Driessen, E., Cuijpers, P., de Maat, S. C., Abbass, A. A., de Jonghe, F., & Dekker, J. J. (2010). The efficacy of short-term psychodynamic psychotherapy for depression: A meta-analysis. *Clinical Psychology Review, 30*(1), 25–36.

Elgersma, H. J., de Jong, P. J., van Rijsbergen, G. D., Kok, G. D., Burger, H., van der Does, W., ... & Bockting, C. L. (2015). Cognitive reactivity, self-depressed associations, and the recurrence of depression. *Journal of Affective Disorders, 183,* 300–309.

Fonagy, P., Rost, F., Carlyle, J. A., McPherson, S., Thomas, R., Pasco Fearon, R. M., ... & Taylor, D. (2015). Pragmatic randomized controlled trial of long-term psychoanalytic psychotherapy for treatment-resistant depression: The Tavistock Adult Depression Study (TADS). *World Psychiatry, 14*(3), 312–321.

Franck, E., De Raedt, R., & De Houwer, J. (2008). Activation of latent self-schemas as a cognitive vulnerability factor for depression: The potential role of implicit self-esteem. *Cognition and Emotion, 22*(8), 1588–1599.

Freud, S. (1917/1957). Mourning and Melancholia. In J. Strachey (Ed.), *The standard edition of the complete psychological works of Sigmund Freud, Volume XIV (1914–1916)* (pp. 237–258). London: The Hogarth Press and the Institute of Psycho-analysis.

Friedmann, J. S., Lumley, M. N., & Lerman, B. (2016). Cognitive schemas as longitudinal predictors of self-reported adolescent depressive symptoms and resilience. *Cognitive Behaviour Therapy, 45*(1), 32–48.

Gotlib, I. H., Krasnoperova, E., Yue, D. N., & Joormann, J. (2004). Attentional biases for negative interpersonal stimuli in clinical depression. *Journal of Abnormal Psychology, 113*(1), 127–139.

Heim, C., Owens, M. J., Plotsky, P. M., & Nemeroff, C. B. (1997). The role of early adverse life events in the etiology of depression and posttraumatic stress disorder. *Annals of the New York Academy of Sciences, 821*(1), 194–207.

Hitchcock, C., Werner-Seidler, A., Blackwell, S. E., & Dalgleish, T. (2017). Autobiographical episodic memory-based training for the treatment of mood, anxiety and stress-related disorders: A systematic review and meta-analysis. *Clinical Psychology Review, 52,* 92–107.

Ingram, B. L. (2011). *Clinical case formulations: Matching the integrative treatment plan to the client.* New York: Wiley.

Jorm, A. F., Christensen, H., Henderson, A. S., Jacomb, P. A., Korten, A. E., & Rodgers, B. (1998). Using the BIS/BAS scales to measure behavioural inhibition and behavioural activation: Factor structure, validity and norms in a large community sample. *Personality and Individual Differences, 26*(1), 49–58.

Kelvin, R. G., Goodyer, I. M., Teasdale, J. D., & Brechin, D. (1999). Latent negative self-schema and high emotionality in well adolescents at risk for psychopathology. *The Journal of Child Psychology and Psychiatry and Allied Disciplines, 40*(6), 959–968.

Kierkegaard, S. (1843/1992). The unhappiest one. In S. Kierkegaard (Ed.), *Either/Or: A fragment of life* (A. Hannair, Trans., pp. 209–222). London: Penguin Classics.

Kroenke, K., Spitzer, R. L., & Williams, J. B. (2001). The PHQ-9: Validity of a brief depression severity measure. *Journal of General Internal Medicine, 16*(9), 606–613.

Kuyken, W., & Brewin, C. R. (1995). Autobiographical memory functioning in depression and reports of early abuse. *Journal of Abnormal Psychology, 104*(4), 585–596.

Laidlaw, K., & Davidson, K. M. (2001). The personal nature of depression: Assessing the operation of self-schema in depression. *Clinical Psychology & Psychotherapy: An International Journal of Theory & Practice, 8*(2), 97–105.

Lau, M. A., Segal, Z. V., & Williams, J. M. G. (2004). Teasdale's differential activation hypothesis: Implications for mechanisms of depressive relapse and suicidal behaviour. *Behaviour Research and Therapy, 42*(9), 1001–1017.

Leichsenring, F. (2001). Comparative effects of short-term psychodynamic psychotherapy and cognitive-behavioral therapy in depression: A meta-analytic approach. *Clinical Psychology Review, 21*(3), 401–419.

Lemogne, C., Bergouignan, L., Piolino, P., Jouvent, R., Allilaire, J. F., & Fossati, P. (2009). Cognitive avoidance of intrusive memories and autobiographical memory: Specificity, autonoetic consciousness, and self-perspective. *Memory, 17*(1), 1–7.

Lemogne, C., Piolino, P., Friszer, S., Claret, A., Girault, N., Jouvent, R., ... & Fossati, P. (2006). Episodic autobiographical memory in depression: Specificity, autonoetic consciousness, and self-perspective. *Consciousness and cognition, 15*(2), 258–268.

Masterson, C., Ekers, D., Gilbody, S., Richards, D., Toner-Clewes, B., & McMillan, D. (2014). Sudden gains in behavioural activation for depression. *Behaviour Research and Therapy, 60*, 34–38.

Paykel, E. S. (2008). Basic concepts of depression. *Dialogues in Clinical Neuroscience, 10*(3), 279–283.

Pinto-Meza, A., Caseras, X., Soler, J., Puigdemont, D., Pérez, V., & Torrubia, R. (2006). Behavioural inhibition and behavioural activation systems in current and recovered major depression participants. *Personality and Individual Differences, 40*(2), 215–226.

Plagnol, A. (2002). Peine, douleur et dépression. *Annales Médico-Psychologiques, 160*, 615–621.

Plagnol, A. (2004). *Espaces de représentation: Théorie élémentaire et psycho-pathologie* [Representational spaces: Elements and psychopathology]. Paris: Editions du CNRS.

Plagnol, A., & Mirabel-Sarron, C. (2006). Schémas dépressogènes et espace subjectif. *Annales Médico-Psychologiques, 164*, 24–33.

Santos, M. M., Rae, J. R., Nagy, G. A., Manbeck, K. E., Hurtado, G. D., West, P., ... & Kanter, J. W. (2017). A client-level session-by-session evaluation of behavioral activation's mechanism of action. *Journal of Behavior Therapy and Experimental Psychiatry, 54*, 93–100.

Seeds, P. M., & Dozois, D. J. (2010). Prospective evaluation of a cognitive vulnerability-stress model for depression: The interaction of schema self-structures and negative life events. *Journal of Clinical Psychology, 66*(12), 1307–1323.

Segal, Z. V. (1988). Appraisal of the self-schema construct in cognitive models of depression. *Psychological Bulletin, 103*(2), 147–178.

Seligman, M. E. (1972). Learned helplessness. *Annual Review of Medicine, 23*(1), 407–412.

Spreng, R. N., Mar, R. A., & Kim, A. S. (2009). The common neural basis of autobiographical memory, prospection, navigation, theory of mind, and the default mode: A quantitative meta-analysis. *Journal of Cognitive Neuroscience, 21*(3), 489–510.

Sullivan, H. S. (2013). *The interpersonal theory of psychiatry*. London: Routledge.

Svoboda, E., McKinnon, M. C., & Levine, B. (2006). The functional neuro-anatomy of autobiographical memory: A meta-analysis. *Neuropsychologia*, *44*(12), 2189–2208.

Tolin, D. F. (2010). Is cognitive-behavioral therapy more effective than other therapies?: A meta-analytic review. *Clinical Psychology Review*, *30*(6), 710–720.

Wade, A., Lemming, O. M., & Hedegaard, K. B. (2002). Escitalopram 10 mg/day is effective and well tolerated in a placebo-controlled study in depression in primary care. *International Clinical Psychopharmacology*, *17*(3), 95–102.

Whalley, M. G., Rugg, M. D., & Brewin, C. R. (2012). Autobiographical memory in depression: An fMRI study. *Psychiatry Research: Neuroimaging*, *201*(2), 98–106.

Williams, J. M., & Broadbent, K. (1986). Autobiographical memory in suicide attempters. *Journal of Abnormal Psychology*, *95*(2), 144–158.

Williams, J. M., Teasdale, J. D., Segal, Z. V., & Soulsby, J. (2000). Mindfulness-based cognitive therapy reduces overgeneral autobiographical memory in formerly depressed patients. *Journal of Abnormal Psychology*, *109*(1), 150–162.

Williams, J. M. G., & Scott, J. (1988). Autobiographical memory in depression. *Psychological Medicine*, *18*(3), 689–695.

Young, J. E., Klosko, J. S., & Weishaar, M. E. (2003). *Schema therapy: A practitioner's guide*. New York: Guilford Press.

7

Traumatic Experiences: When the Home Collapses

1   Introduction

Since their rediscovery during the Vietnam War, post-traumatic stress disorder (PTSD) has become a pillar of contemporary psychopathology, becoming even the keystone of an entire class of disorders in the DSM-5 (American Psychiatric Association, 2013). According to the World Mental Health surveys, lifetime prevalence varies across countries from 1.3% (Japan) to 8.8% (Northern Ireland) (Atwoli, Stein, Koenen, & McLaughlin, 2015). The frequency may be underestimated, particularly because of some complex clinical expressions, for example, in the elderly (Delrue & Plagnol, 2016).

However, in all typical cases, the exposure to a specific event—theatre of war, attack, aggression, rape, fire, accident—causes a disruption of life with deleterious consequences, which often nothing in the previous personality would have predicted. The existence of a *re-experiencing syndrome,* i.e. the almost identical reliving of the traumatic scene, constitutes a remarkable clinical constant. Severity is related to the progressive extension of the functional impact of symptoms: although the starting point is often an isolated event, the subject's entire life can be gradually altered.

© The Author(s) 2019   **131**
T. Ward and A. Plagnol, *Cognitive Psychodynamics as an Integrative
Framework in Counselling Psychology and Psychotherapy,*
https://doi.org/10.1007/978-3-030-25823-8_7

The neurobiological and cognitive mechanisms underlying the re-experiencing syndrome are increasingly understood, which has led to the development of effective therapeutic techniques: Prolonged Exposure (PE) (Foa, Hembree, & Rothbaum, 2007), Eye Movement Desensitization and Reprocessing (EMDR) (Shapiro, 2018), Cognitive Processing Therapy (CPT) (Resick & Schnicke, 1993), Narrative Exposure Therapy (Schauer, Neuner, & Elbert, 2011). However, the processes involved in the triggering of such a syndrome in a given person remain enigmatic, and the most severe forms can pose difficult therapeutic problems (Lehrner, Pratchett, & Yehuda, 2016; Najavits, 2015). The consideration of the inner worlds, building on the development of neurocognitive tools to better describe them, makes it possible to propose new ways to solve these problems (Ward, Plagnol, & Delrue, 2017).

This chapter is therefore an opportunity to introduce in more detail the construction of an inner world and its vicissitudes. First, we will show that the main models of understanding PTSD cannot solve the clinical enigmas raised by these disorders because of the lack of a precise approach to the inner worlds. We will then present an outline of the framework of *representational spaces* that allows such an approach through building on advances in cognitive science. We will show how to solve the enigmas raised by PTSD in this framework, before specifying some new directions opened by cognitive psychodynamics to enrich the methods of treating PTSD.

2   Clinical Enigmas

Let us recall that a psycho-traumatic disorder is triggered following a situation ("traumatic scene") exposing the subject to the possibility of death or a serious threat to well-being (mutilation, sexual violence…). The main clinical elements are (Lehrner et al., 2016; Plagnol, 2002a):

1. re-experiencing syndrome: reliving of the traumatic scene, flashbacks (images reproducing the situation), intrusive memories;
2. avoidance of stimuli associated with the traumatic scene with hyperarousal towards them;

3. negative alterations in cognition and mood, numbing of emotional relationships, withdrawal from activities, personality changes.

At the time of the traumatic event, a dissociative reaction is the most characteristic clinical expression, but such an acute reaction must be distinguished from the development of a persistent disorder marked by a re-experiencing syndrome. In fact, there is always a delay between the traumatic event and the beginning of a true re-experiencing syndrome.[1] Moreover, up to 25% of cases have a "delayed onset"—at least six months in the DSM-5—often years after the initial event, which current models cannot explain (Bryant, O'Donnell, Creamer, McFarlane, & Silove, 2013; Delrue & Plagnol, 2017).

(From Plagnol, 1991)

Mr A, 32 years old, married and the father of two young children, is hospitalized after being found in the street crying and "delirious".
Mr A's life seemed quiet until a traffic accident a few months earlier, with no physical consequences but which had destroyed his car. A few days after the accident, Mr A became irritable and insomniac, with recurring nightmares. His emotional relationships with family and friends deteriorated, he had to stop working.

During his hospitalization, Mr A constantly refers to the "accident", but it is not the recent traffic accident. Mr A is in fact tormented by a tragic event that occurred fifteen years earlier when he was 17 years old. During a forest trip, a World War I shell exploded, killing three of his friends. Apart from a few nightmares that quickly resolved at the time, young A seemed to have overcome the ordeal well, successfully completing brilliant studies. Mr A now seems to be completely caught up in the revival of this drama: he never ceases to evoke the bloody scene that feeds his nightmares and gets absorbed in existential ruminations that burden his entire social and emotional life.

---

[1]The PTSD in the DSM-5 can only be diagnosed after one month. The acute stress disorder diagnosis does not adequately identify people who develop PTSD (Bryant, 2011).

2.1   Five Enigmas

The existence of PTSD seems to defy the ordinary laws of memory, to the point of raising a series of enigmas (Plagnol, 2004; Ward et al., 2017):

- *The enigma of re-experiencing.* The traumatic scene gives rise to flashbacks and intrusive images that reproduce almost identically the initial percept: How can a memory escape the usual phenomena of decline and reconstruction?
- *The enigma of the extension.* Why, starting from a circumscribed event—the confrontation with a (often) unique scene—do the symptoms end up dominating the whole mental life?
- *The enigma of the delayed action.* There is a delay between the traumatic event and the onset of the re-experiencing syndrome (sometimes several years). How can an event act remotely over time?
- *The enigma of death.* Why confrontation with death (or a threat to bodily integrity) is always involved in triggering a PTSD and causes such severe pathologies when death is as frequent as life (every living being is by definition mortal)?
- *The enigma of vulnerability.* Why does confrontation with the traumatic scene trigger a disorder *only* in some people even if it is something experienced by *many*?[2]

The solutions to these puzzles are often circular, for example, when trying to characterize the traumatic event by indicating that it is "of an exceptionally threatening or catastrophic nature" (World Health Organization, 1992). In addition, as we will now see, the main models that have tried to address post-traumatic stress disorders fail to take into account *all* of these enigmas.

---

[2]15–25% of people facing trauma develop PTSD (Lehrner et al., 2016).

2.2   Limitations of Classic Models

Let us take as a starting point the model of Foa, which is at the origin of the cognitive-behavioural reference therapies for PTSD. In this model, the representation of the traumatic event would be associated with a *fear structure* in memory (Foa, Steketee, & Rothbaum, 1989), i.e. a network of memory units encoding the event, the person's reaction and the meaning associated to them. When a traumatic syndrome is triggered, the "basic safety rules" would be violated, so that "one's world becomes less predictable and controllable" (p. 166). Based also on the principles of conditioning, such a model partly accounts for the enigmas of re-experiencing, extension and delayed action.

But why does the traumatic scene induce the presence of a fear structure? What does a safe and predictable world mean from a psychological point of view? Why do only some individuals have their basic beliefs broken in such a situation? If the meaning of the event is not taken into account (as in purely behaviourist approaches), it is impossible to answer such questions; but if the threatening meaning of the event is highlighted, the answer is circular—unless one specifies what "safe" and "predictable" means in relation to the individual's inner world.

In a more psychodynamic framework, Horowitz (1986, 1990) explicitly took into account the upheaval of the world by the traumatic event: by hitting the basic beliefs of the individual, the traumatic scene could not be integrated into the individual's "world model"—in other words, his/her inner world—hence, a process of defence by denial; therefore, because of a "principle of completion" requiring the integration of any event into the world model, the traumatic scene would remain active and generate intrusions in consciousness.

Janoff-Bulman also considers that the traumatic event causes an upheaval of the inner world by shattering fundamental assumptions about the world (Janoff-Bulman, 1992; Janoff-Bulman & McPherson Franz, 1997). Her work takes some important steps to clarify what "a safe and predictable world" means: at the core of our inner world, we would have "working models" about ourselves and about the outer world, notably that the outer world is meaningful and controllable by our action. However, such fundamental assumptions are general abstract beliefs, and Janoff-Bulman does not propose a detailed construction of the inner world, nor does she specify the elementary representational and memory processes that underlie the "meaning-making" that seems so essential to our lives and so hurt in PTSD.

In particular, it still remains to be explained why a life-threatening experience disrupts the fundamental assumptions of the subject. A psychoanalytical response could be attempted on this point: according to Freud (1915/1957), the unconscious operates with a postulate of immortality, so it is impossible for us to really represent our own death (we can only imagine it by remaining a spectator). But *how does what we cannot represent have such deleterious effects on the inner world, whilst the inner world is constituted from representations?* We are brought back to the need to develop a precise approach to the construction of an inner world as well as a full analysis of the interaction of a traumatic event with memory.

2.3   On the Neurosciences Side

Neuroscience-inspired models of PTSD today focus on the impairments of *episodic memory* (that is, the memory of situations in space and time[3]). In short, exposition to the traumatic scene would trigger such an intense emotion that the amygdalian circuit is overactivated and hippocampal structures impaired (Bremner, 2006; Lehrner et al., 2016; Samuelson, 2011; Sherin & Nemeroff, 2011), whilst these structures normally have a key role in episodic memory (Moscovitch, Cabeza, Winocur, & Nadel, 2016). The integration of the traumatic experience would thus be interrupted (van der Kolk, 2000), with possible dissociative symptoms. From then on, the scene would tend to return unchanged in consciousness—that is, to be re-experienced—resulting in an emotion that is still as intense as ever, with an overactivation of the amygdala once again, and a repetition of the dissociative reaction.

Such a model provides a fairly good account of the re-experiencing enigma and effectiveness of the trauma-focused therapies (PE, EMDR, etc.),

---

[3]See Chapters 2 and 4.

which are often considered to be "gold standard" PTSD therapies (see Najavits, 2015). What these therapies have in common is that they try to reduce the emotional intensity caused by the evocation of the traumatic scene, so that the client can resume the mental work on this scene, for example, by writing a scenario in which he/she regains control of the situation, and can finally integrate the scene in a peaceful way into his/her inner world.

However, the other puzzles raised by PTSD remain intact. Why can the traumatic scene trigger such an intense emotion? Why do certain effects take so long to manifest themselves, but eventually weigh on the whole life? Why does the presence of death or the violation of integrity have such deleterious effects? Why are only certain individuals affected?

Moreover, the "gold standard" therapies have certain limitations: some PTSD are resistant to these techniques, relapses are observed or there is a substantial dropout in real-world practice (Najavits, 2015). This is particularly true when PTSD is severe; for example, an intense dissociative reaction or a fear of distress can be a barrier to trauma-focused therapy (Fareng & Plagnol, 2014; Lehrner et al., 2016). In addition, these therapies focus on the re-experiencing syndrome, but in severe cases, it is necessary to be able to address the impact of the disorder on the subject's entire existence. Cognitive therapies such as CPT address the belief schemas that sustain PTSD and propose cognitive restructuring to modify the meaning attributed to the traumatic event, but a more thorough consideration of psychosocial factors, existential impact on the inner world and "search for meaning" is sometimes necessary (Alim et al., 2008; Iacoviello & Charney, 2016; Janoff-Bulman & McPherson Franz, 1997).

3 Contributions of the Model Proposed by Brewin

Taking into account the limitations of previous models, particularly those of Foa and Horowitz, Brewin and his colleagues have proposed a particularly refined model of post-traumatic stress disorder (Brewin, Dalgleish, & Joseph, 1996; Brewin, Gregory, Lipton, & Burgess, 2010).

This model also highlights the key role of episodic memory but is based on a precise theory of mental representations, which makes it possible to exploit a striking feature of intrusive representations of the traumatic scene, namely that they are "percept-like" and reproduce almost exactly the original scene.

3.1   Dual Representation Theory and Its Neural Bases

Brewin and his colleagues' first proposed *dual representation theory* (Brewin et al., 1996), by borrowing from cognitive psychology an essential distinction between two types of representations:

- some are "situational", i.e. *analogical,* quasi-sensory (perceptual or image-like) and implicit;
- the others are of a verbal type, i.e. *symbolic,* explicit and accessible to the conscience[4];

The mnemonic integration of an event presupposes that symbolic representations are associated with its situational representation, which makes it possible to give it a meaning for consciousness. This process can be interrupted ("premature inhibition", according to Brewin et al.) if the beliefs that underlie the inner world—for example, the belief that the universe makes sense—are incompatible with the event. A traumatic syndrome occurs when the situational representation of an event remains active without its symbolic processing being completed.

Brewin et al. (2010) redesigned this model and clarified the neural bases of both types of representation: sensory representations (S-representations) depend on the temporo-occipital and parietal cortex, as well as the amygdala (dorsal flux); symbolic representations (C-representations) depend on the mediotemporal cortex and the hippocampus (ventral flux). C-representations ensure the contextualization

---

[4]The analogical/symbolic terminology is more ours than that of Brewin et al. We are following a well-established tradition in cognitive science (e.g. Plagnol, 2004).

of S-representations and thus allow the integration of an event in episodic memory. Moreover, some connections between the prefrontal cortex and the mediotemporal cortex provide specific retrieval cues to episodic representations. In this way, C-representations can give a meaningful interpretation of an event (that was initially represented in S-memory).

PTSD would occur in cases of "extreme stress" associated with a feeling of "mental defeat" leading to impaired hippocampal functioning. In such a case, S-representations could not be associated with C-representations. As a result, the event would not be integrated into episodic memory and would remain active in its "S-rep" form. Moreover, active S-representations can be automatically triggered by associated stimuli, which will result in the phenomenon of "flashbacks", themselves a source of avoidance of everything that can trigger them because of their "unpleasant" character.

3.2 Some Limits of the Brewin Model

Brewin's model provides a better understanding of the effectiveness of "gold standard therapies" (such as PE or EMDR): as noted, they are based on resuming the mental work on the traumatic scene through the control of the emotional reaction, which can be understood as the association of C-representations to S-representations—in other words, the subject successfully associates symbolic (verbal) representations with mental imagery representing the traumatic scene, hence, its integration into episodic memory.

However, the explanation of PTSD remains circular: why does the event that causes PTSD lead to "extreme stress" and "mental defeat"? Why is a flashback of the event "unpleasant"? In addition, why do particular events trigger PTSD in some people and not others? How can an event resonate with a singular story? A better understanding of the interaction between an event and a unique subjective memory can be essential for clinical work.

(After Delrue & Plagnol, 2016)

Mrs W, 97 years old, enters a retirement home and quickly suffers severe pain in her right arm, which is medically unexplained despite a complete check-up. She also complains of stomach aches and hyperphagia for sweet foods. In addition, Mrs W is hyper-vigilant: she watches for the slightest noise and the slightest coming. Finally, Mrs W shows an important avoidance: fatigue justifies retreating to her room and sleep allows her to escape the pain.

A precise analysis of Mrs W's story reveals an old trauma. Indeed, during World War I, when she was 5 years old, Mrs W's father died with his arm torn off. She was then raised by a mother without resources and was malnourished.

The psychological assessment confirms the co-occurrence of PTSD. The psychologist hypothesizes that the pain presented by Mrs W since entering the retirement home is related to the trauma that remained silent for many years, as suggested by the possible link between her severe arm pain and her father's tragic death. In addition, stomach aches and eating disorders could be related to food deprivation during the war. (Mrs W was eating candy hidden in a tin can.)

The psychologist decides to treat pain and PTSD simultaneously, at a pace appropriate to Mrs W's age and resources, which is two sessions per week for 10 weeks. First, Mrs W is asked to focus on her somatic sensations, describe her painful experience and indicate whether she has experienced similar pains in the past. Joint work is then undertaken on PTSD and chronic pain. Mrs W externalizes and reworks the emotions associated with the traumatic scene. The work on chronic pain relies on relaxation to help Mrs W feel, identify, and describe the painful sensations. The links between the painful sensations and the trauma are discussed.

At the end of the therapy, there is a complete disappearance of PTSD, pain and symptoms. At six months, the recovery is stable, and Mrs W has resumed activities in the retirement home.

The turning point of Mrs W's case was the psychologist's hypothesis that there was a resonance between her unexplainable pain in her right arm and her earlier story, which was probably reactivated when she entered an institution. The detection of such resonance is not possible with brain imaging techniques! Mrs W's sense of pain could only be understood by an intimate approach to her lived history, that is, by an encounter with her inner world.

In summary, what we need in a case like Mrs W's is the intimate focus that a psychotherapeutic encounter can offer, which can take into account the meaning of the traumatic event in relation to the person's inner world, in order to define a "tailor-made" care protocol.

4   Representational Spaces and Traumatic Events

Let us summarize what seems necessary for a refined approach to traumatic syndromes:

1. specify the modalities of the integration of an event into the inner world (and the hazards preventing such an integration); in particular, in accordance with Brewin's model, to have a detailed theory of the mental work on an event as a transition from an analogue/perceptual format of representation to a symbolic/verbal format;
2. account for the meaning of the traumatic event in relation to the person's inner world, as it can be shaped by his or her history recorded in memory.

The approach of the inner world as a representational space (Plagnol, 2002b, 2004, in press) allows these objectives to be met. Indeed, this approach proposes a construction of the inner world as it can be deployed from memory, building on the duality between analogical and symbolic representations. In fact, *this duality is explained precisely by the need to construct an inner world from a limited window of presence.*

To understand this, let us take the time to sketch out the construction of an inner world as a representational space. Then, equipped with such tools, we will come back to traumatic situations and their impact on such a space.

4.1   Representational Bases

In our conceptual framework, the inner world is considered as the unified set of contents accessible by the mental system of representation—in other words, the inner world is constituted as a *representational space*.

However, as we saw in Chapter 2, the focus of conscious attention or presence window defined by the global workspace is very limited. In particular, the content that can be deployed at any given time in the conscious workspace (or *work plan* [Plagnol, 2004, in press])—in conjunction with processes such as the *visuospatial sketchpad* (Baddeley, 1986), *spatial array* (Ragni & Knauff, 2013), *spatial field* (Lyon, Gunzelmann, & Gluck, 2008), etc.[5]—is limited: only a very tiny part of an individual's representational space is deployed at any given time.

- *Analogical* (or *situational*) *representations* can be defined as elementary fragments of representation that directly deploy content in the work plan: perceptions from current experience or more or less abstract projections from memory (e.g. mental images [Kosslyn, Thompson, & Ganis, 2006] or mental models [Johnson-Laird, 1983]).

Since the analogical representations are closely limited by the boundaries of the presence window, developing complex or extended content requires the possibility of unifying such representations by dynamically linking them in the work plan, that is, it requires "navigating" in the representational space (as one navigates the Internet by linking contents in the computer's browser window). Such navigation also requires the ability to store in memory representations that are not deployed in the work plan (just as the contents of websites that are not deployed in the browser window are stored in a memory.[6])

- *Symbolic representations* make it possible to code analogical representations, store them in memory in a reduced format and link them in the work plan when they are reactivated (like web pages are linked by hypertext links).

---

[5]See Chapter 2 on the capacity limitations of working memory. The work plan can be conceived as the main component of the workspace through which contents are displayed. Such a deployment component could be understood as largely spatial and supra-modal, as studies of spatial representations of blind subjects suggest (Afonso et al., 2010; Giudice, Betty, & Loomis, 2011).

[6]This comparison between mental navigation and web browsing will be extended in Chapter 9.

- The symbolic units are associated by links that reflect the previous experience of the subject: their whole constitutes the *symbolic web* of the representational space.

The millions of analogical fragments formed during a singular history can thus be integrated in *one* inner world thanks to the symbolic web. Only a small part of the symbolic web is active at any given time. The activation flow is a function of the stimulations of the experience and the associative links. The *tension* exerted on a representational space can be considered as mirroring its complexity, i.e. as an inverse function of its degree of unification/consistency/congruence.[7] The basic principle describing the associative flow of representations is a Principle of Unification: the representational system constantly tends to minimize tension on the active part of the representational space, which amounts to trying to unify it.

> The Principle of Unification can be compared to Horowitz's Completion Principle (Horowitz, 1990). Such a principle is found in many forms and conceptual frameworks (e.g. Clark, 2013, pp. 186–187; Conway, Singer, & Tagini, 2004; Freud, 1915/1990; Grawe, 2007). It can be considered as a psychological application of the Principle of Least Action: according to Shepard (2008), the Principle of Least Action not only underlies any process in nature, but can also be derived a priori from fundamental principles of transformation and symmetry.

New sources of tension are constantly created by the flow of external and internal events that generate new analogical representations (perceptions, mental images, mental models...) in the work plan. Indeed, an event implies a change in the work plan, with a modification of the active web. The symbolic processing of an event, through automatic processes of symbolic association or through processes of conscious analysis, makes it possible in principle to transform an

---

[7]Remember the importance of the notions of consistency and congruence highlighted in Chapters 3–5.

analogical representation into a symbolic web fragment encoding the essential aspects of the event and ensuring its integration into the inner world, in accordance with the Principle of Unification.

4.2   Impact of a Traumatic Situation

Let us now introduce some concepts to account accurately for a traumatic interaction between an event and a representational space:

- A *conflict* is an incompatibility between fragments of the work plan, which induces a point of tension, which must be resolved according to the Principle of Unification.
- A *defence process* is a solution to a conflict such that one of the conflict fragments is unloaded from the work plan without being fully processed. (This corresponds to the notion of premature inhibition of Brewin et al., 1996.)
- Due to the Principle of Unification, an analogical fragment that isn't fully processed remains active outside the work plan, becoming an *interfering fragment*.
- A traumatic sequence can then be described:

  - An event triggers an analogical representation A that is deployed in the work plan;
  - A is analysed by the symbolic processes and a web fragment W is gradually associated with it;
  - Some elements of W reactivate by association a fragment W' of the web;
  - W' causes a projection of an analogical fragment A' in the work plan;
  - A and A' are incompatible and conflict;
  - A is removed from the active plan before it has been completely processed ("premature inhibition");
  - A becomes an interfering fragment;
  - A is a source of significant tensions, not having been integrated into the inner world. According to the Principle of Unification, A tends to intrude into the work plan.

Mr B is attacked in the parking lot of his bank by a man with a gun: "Your wallet!". As Mr B clumsily searches his coat, the man points the gun at his head. Once the wallet is handed over, the man disappears.

Some time later, Mr B developed a severe post-traumatic stress disorder. He constantly reviews the scene of the attack, in particular the movement of the revolver in the man's hand: "It was a beautiful revolver...". Mr B explains that he had the vision of his wife and children hearing the news of his death whilst they were waiting for him like every evening for dinner. Every time he reviews the scene of the attack, it is associated with the image of the family dinner and Mr B breaks down in tears.

If we analyse the traumatic sequence with the tools we have introduced, the event is the aggression, the analogical representation A is the scene with the revolver. It can be assumed that symbolic units such as *revolver, blood, death*, are activated when processing this scene. By association, items such as *mourning, family, home, dinner*, are in turn activated. The projection A' of a family dinner scene hit the scene A of the attack. The tension being too intense, A is removed from the work plan. Since A could not be processed, it remains active, interfering with the content deployed in the work plan. Because of the Principle of Unification, the scene A tends to return intrusively in Mr B's presence window, but the same phenomenon occurs: the conflict between A and a scene of family happiness always leads to early inhibition of A's symbolic process.

The more traumatic a representation is, the more quickly its symbolic processing is inhibited and the more it tends to intrude in its initial form, close to perceptual processes if it is a percept. In PTSD, the quasi-perceptual reproduction of the traumatic scene shows that it is stored in memory in a superficial form. An intense conflict thus occurs between this scene and other fragments of the representational space, at an early stage of the scene's symbolic processing, resulting in a dissociative defence, preventing its integration into the inner world and causing the "eternal return of the same".

4.3   The Progressive Extension of the Traumatic Grip

The enigma of repetition is therefore handled in our framework in essentially the same terms as in Brewin's model, namely early symbolic inhibition. However, our meaning-oriented perspective, by taking into account the meaning of an event in relation to the inner world, will also allow us to account for the progressive extension of the impact of PTSD on the inner world, i.e. to tackle the enigmas of extension and delayed action we have raised in Sect. 2.1.

Let's come back to the case of Mr B who saw too close a too beautiful gun. During the first few weeks, Mr B seemed to overcome the violent aggression he suffered. He was able to file a complaint with the police and resumed his work the next day. However, he kept talking about the attack, started having nightmares, then became irritable, angry, ruminating endlessly about the scene in the bank's parking lot where his life was brutally in danger.

Mr B had to stop working and embarked on endless efforts to obtain compensation, despairing of what he considered to be a failure of society towards him. His family life has been deeply affected by his recent intolerance to the slightest conflict, his violent outbursts of anger, his life's focus on aggression and his attempts to obtain a "fair compensation". According to Mr B, "everything is wrong at home" and his life "no longer makes sense". Traditional therapies (drugs, cognitive-behavioural approaches) do little to help him overcome this feeling that now permeates his entire life.

The traumatic event eventually came into conflict with the whole of Mr B's inner world, despite his willingness to fight against what was invading him. How has such an extension gradually developed?

4.3.1 The Paradigm of Traumatic Mourning

A misfortune is all the more difficult to symbolically process in a complete way when it is incompatible with large areas of the representational space. For example, a romantic break-up is all the more long to process when large areas of the space of the person who is in love are associated with the loved one and incompatible with the break-up.

We find here in fact the psychodynamic notion of "work of mourning" advanced by Freud in *Mourning and Melancholy* (1917/1957). According to this famous text, when a loved one is lost, a slow process of symbolic work is necessary to overcome the suffering of loss, because each memory or project conflicts with this loss and generates a wave of pain.

In our conceptual framework, a work of mourning involves confronting the reality of loss with each fragment of the representational space associated with the lost person, which requires a reworking of the entire space when the lost person has been installed at the heart of the inner world. Some bereavements can be associated with PTSD, especially in the event of a sudden confrontation with the dying body of a loved one.[8]

> Mrs X, 55, comes to see a psychologist because she is not recovering from her husband's death. With a motor disability since childhood, she met her husband late, but experienced intense happiness for twelve years: "He was everything to me". Unfortunately, her husband died suddenly from an aneurysm rupture that nothing could have predicted. He collapsed on the carpet in their living room and Mrs X could only lie next to him whilst waiting for help. Since then, she has been constantly reviewing this scene where she lies near her husband's body, the arrival of the emergency services, the vain attempts at resuscitation. Mrs X blames herself for not having been able to save her husband; since then, "the home is empty", her life "no longer makes sense".

As the loss of her companion touched the heart of Mrs X's space—both mental and physical since her husband died on the carpet of her living room where she spends all day because of her disability—the revolver on Mr B's temple must have struck central pillars of his inner world.

---

[8]"Complicated" or "complex and persistent" bereavement tends to be considered as a pathological entity since the DSM-5 for which it is a proposed diagnosis for further studies. According to Shear and Gribbin (2016), complex and persistent bereavement must be distinguished from PTSD, which follows exposure to a danger (while complex and persistent bereavement is induced by the loss of a highly invested relative). However, a bereavement can be linked with PTSD if it involves a confrontation with the scene of death (and the dying body of the loved one becoming a corpse) before a re-experiencing syndrome. You can compare such a bereavement with PTSD to Sarah's case in Chapter 4: Sarah's brother's accidental death resulted in unresolved grief for her, but without PTSD. (It could have been different if Sarah had been present at the accident.) Those who like diagnostic labels would probably talk about "persistent complex bereavement" in Sarah's case. It should be noted that her grief, even without being associated to a PTSD, is nevertheless traumatic in a sense that our conceptual framework makes it possible to specify (see the concluding remarks of this chapter).

4.3.2 Ideal of the Home and Loss of Meaning

Although they both live in a confined apartment, both Mrs X and Mr B refer to the collapse of their "home". Indeed, as we already suggested in Chapter 6, the inner world is often organized according to a fundamental intuition, which we can call the ideal of *the Home*, associated with an ideal house projection where family happiness can unfold without clouds (Plagnol, 2004). In the case of Mr B as in the case of Mrs X, the loss of the Home is correlated to a meaningless life.

In our conceptual framework, a "loss of meaning" is specified as an impossibility of deploying a unified space. A traumatic event actually hits the Principle of Unification that underlies any representation: not only does the traumatic event give rise to a conflict, but this conflict is prolonged in an intuition of its irremediable nature, with no hope of a solution. From then on, any project seems impossible to be unified with the traumatic scene; similarly, the past history becomes retrospectively failed, because it cannot be unified with this scene. In particular, there is no longer a possible scenario for achieving the Home ideal: the world will never be reconciled.

The conflict may at first seem local and solvable: the subject may seem to accept the event, sometimes in the form of a struggle, as was the case in the first weeks for Mr B. But this apparent acceptance is only defensive: the traumatic scene has been removed from the work plan without being processed in depth; not integrated into the inner world, this scene comes back to intrude and conflicts with a new fragment of the subjective space; as this conflict proves insoluble again, a defence still interrupts the process of the traumatic scene, and the cycle repeats itself.

Thus, the traumatic scene is gradually associated with every representation, up to the point where it settles at the centre of the inner world, that is, it is associated with every zone of the subjective space, like a poison that has infiltrated the body with each round of circulation and eventually reached the heart (Plagnol, 2002a).

4.4   Death and Ruin of the Home

Why does an event cause a loss of meaning? A fundamental characteristic of traumatic events is to face death directly (as is the case for Mrs X), or to constitute an imminent threat of death (as for Mr B), or to ruin the daily space of the house (flood, fire, brutal news of the death of a family member, etc.).

In any case, a scene directly contradicts the ideal of the Home, which allows ordinary events to be integrated, and this without any projectable reconstruction. In particular, death implies not only the definitive deprivation of life, but also confronts the unknown of the "after", without possible representation, therefore without possible meaning, except through spiritual beliefs (which in some cases are a protective factor against PTSD [Briant-Davis & Wong, 2013; Hourani et al., 2012; Iacoviello & Charney, 2016; Slater, Bordenave, & Boyer, 2016]).

The shock of losing a child who has grown up in the heart of the Home often destroys the intimate meaning of life (Shear & Gribbin, 2016). The great French romantic poet, Alphonse de Lamartine, suffered such an intolerable trauma when his 10-year-old daughter Julia died in his arms in Beirut on 7 December 1832 (see Plagnol, 2014). In his poem *Gethsemani ou la mort de Julia* [*Gethsmane or Julia's Death*] (1835/2001), Lamartine re-experiences the moment his inner world collapsed:

Et je sentis ainsi, dans une heure éternelle,
Passer des mers d'angoisse et des siècles d'horreur,
Et la douleur combla la place où fut mon cœur[9];

The poet's inner world is directly identified with the lost child:

C'était mon univers, mon mouvement, mon bruit,
La voix qui m'enchantait dans toutes mes demeures
Le charme ou le souci de mes yeux, de mes heures,
Mon matin, mon soir et ma nuit![10]

The ruin of the Home is expressed with a heartbreaking accent:

Maintenant tout est mort dans ma maison aride,
Deux yeux toujours pleurant sont toujours devant moi[11]

---

[9] *And I felt in an eternal hour/Passing seas of anguish and centuries of horror/And the pain filled the place where my heart was;* (our translation).

[10] *It was my world, my movement, my sound,/The voice that enchanted me in all my homes/The charm or concern of my eyes, my hours/My morning, my evening and my night!*

[11] *Now everything is dead in my dried home/Two eyes ever crying stand ever before me.*

Only the poet's faith opens a door to a possible meaning:

> *Mais c'est Dieu qui t'écrase, ô mon âme! sois forte,*
> *Baise sa main sous la douleur!*[12]

Lamartine's poetic breath, then 42 years old, dries up around this time. However, at 66 years old, returning to his native house that needed to be sold, he found a dazzling inspiration to write his "swan song", La Vigne et la Maison [*The Vine and the Home*] (1857/2001):

> *Efface ce séjour, ô Dieu! de ma paupière,*
> *Ou rends-le-moi semblable à celui d'autrefois,*
> *Quand la maison vibrait comme un grand cœur de pierre*
> *De tous ces cœurs joyeux qui battaient sous ses toits!*[13]

4.5   Vulnerability

Even if the nature of certain events, such as direct confrontation with death, may hit the assumptions that underlie the inner world in most individuals, the development of a traumatic syndrome depends on the interaction of this scene with the singular history written in subjective memory.

The possibility of an existential upheaval depends on the previous experiences of the person confronted with the traumatic event. We had mentioned about Mrs W, the resonance between her painful arm at the entrance to the retirement home and her father's arm torn off during the war. Similarly, Lamartine's poem, *The Vine and the Home*, resonates with all the bereavements that struck the poet.[14] And for Mrs X, her husband's mourning revives the loss of her parents and the burden of her disability, the existential impact being all the more severe as she finds herself physically very vulnerable and unprotected.

---

[12]*But it is God who crushes you, O my soul!/Be strong, kiss His hand under the pain!*

[13]*Erase this stay, O God! from my eyelid,/Or make it like the one it used to be/When the Home vibrated like a big heart of stone/All those happy hearts beating under his roof!*

[14]Beside the death of his daughter Julia in 1831, Lamartine had experienced many other close bereavements, including the tragic death of Julie Charles in 1817 with whom he had a passionate romance. (It is disturbing to note that Lamartine's first major collection of poems, *Méditations poétiques* [*Poetic Meditations*] [1820/2001], considered to be the moment of birth of French romantic poetry, was published shortly after the death of Julie Charles, who largely inspired it.)

The solidity of the foundations of the inner world is crucial to over-coming traumatic experiences, in particular the coherence of the "child-hood space" defined by the parental images and representations of the childhood house, the school, the hometown, etc. Past traumas, not fully integrated into the inner world, constitute on the contrary areas of vul-nerability (Bryant et al., 2013; Delrue & Plagnol, 2016, 2017). When the onset of a traumatic syndrome seems inexplicable, the exploration of the singular history most often leads to the discovery of old traumas that are not sufficiently symbolically processed (see the case of Mr A at the beginning of this chapter).

Overprotection in childhood may also increase vulnerability in adult-hood. In such a case, we often find an idealized parental home—this is the case for Mr B who desperately compares the collapse of his home to the security of his childhood home.

5   Inner Worlds and PTSD Therapy

Table 1 summarizes the explanations provided by our conceptual frame-work to the enigmas raised by traumatic syndromes.

By allowing for a better understanding of the devastating disrup-tions of the inner world, representational spaces provide an integra-tive framework for "tailor-made" adjustment of therapeutic objectives and methods, as is intended in the cognitive-psychodynamic approach

Table 1 Explanation of five enigmas set up by post-traumatic stress disorders

Enigma	Explanation
Re-experiencing	The traumatic scene stays represented within an analogical (situational) representational format, without being trans-formed in a symbolic format
Extension	The traumatic scene stirs up an incompatibility reaction with any other memory reactivated
Delay	The traumatic scene needs time to "infect" the inner world
Death	The traumatic scene hits the foundations of the inner world like the Home ideal
Vulnerability	The effect of the traumatic scene depends on its resonance with the personal story as it has shaped the inner world

we advocate here. We outline below some ways to develop such a perspective.

- Taking into account the inner worlds of clients allows us to better justify the methods that have proven their efficacy in most PTSD by curing the syndrome of re-experiencing (PR, EMDR, CPT...). Indeed, their common point is to help the person to resume the symbolic work on a life-threatening or other traumatic experience interrupted by a strong emotion of distress. A precise approach to the interaction between the traumatic event and the inner world should make it possible to better locate the critical point where symbolic work has been interrupted ("premature inhibition", according to Brewin et al., 1996), as well as the extent and specificity of the cognitive restructuring necessary to integrate the event into the inner world and restore a coherent life story.
- In severe cases of PTSD associated with comorbidities, resistance to standard therapies, or relapse after the use of reference techniques, treatment of the re-experiencing syndrome alone is insufficient, due to the existential impact of PTSD, but also to a vulnerability whose roots are buried in the subject's past.

In such cases, a more phenomenological, existential or psychodynamic approach may be beneficial to complement therapies that are effective for the re-experiencing syndrome, even if it may require a longer treatment period. In accordance with the seminal works of Horowitz and Janoff-Bulman, and more recent studies that highlight the importance of the meaning-making process in the recovery (e.g. Alim et al., 2008), the therapy may be directed towards supporting the person to recover a meaningful universe that integrates the trauma, which a more systematic approach to the inner world, based on the tools developed in cognitive science, can now facilitate, hence, the interest of cognitive psychodynamics here.

In Table 2, we list some basic points that the therapist can evaluate before moving in this direction with the client, including the very important point of also considering his/her own inner world.

Table 2 First steps towards exploring the inner world in PTSD from the perspective of cognitive psychodynamics

Explore the client's inner world

– Look for the spatial metaphors used by the client for family and professional life ("life course", "path", "home", etc.), disease ("no way out", "darkness", etc.), therapeutic encounter ("support", etc.);

– What do these metaphors reflect about his/her inner world?

– Are there basic beliefs and fundamental assumptions that underlie these metaphors?—Are there any conceptions of life and death involved?

– Is the client's inner world unified? Is there a keystone that gives meaning to life?

– Is it possible to use these metaphors with the client to make him/her aware of some essential features of his/her own inner world?

– What precautions should be taken?

– What are the links between the inner world and its environment ("outer" world)?

– Was the outer world safe and predictable before the traumatic event?

Explore the effects of the traumatic event on the inner world

– How could one describe the incongruence between the traumatic scene and the inner world?

– How can the client describe the changes that the traumatic event has produced in his or her inner world?

– Does the client feel that basic beliefs have been disrupted?

– Does the client feel a loss of ideal? A loss of safety? A loss of meaning?

– What moves or blocking points are suggested by his/her emotions?

– Is a re-experiencing syndrome still active?

– Is there an experience of low mood or depression? If so, what impact does it have on the inner world?

– How does the client feel about the therapeutic space between his/her inner world and the outer world? Is he/she in a safe place?

Resonances with the past

– Are there some detectable resonances between the traumatic event and past events?

– Does the subject spontaneously evoke older traumatic events? What time did they come back? Are they still active? What have been their effects on the inner world? What are the symbolic links with the current traumatic event?

– Are there any other less prominent traumatic event that can be identified?

– What hypotheses can be made about the "roots" of the vulnerability? Does the client evoke these spontaneously?

– How to characterize the childhood Home? Was it a safe and predictable place?

– How to characterize the parental figures in childhood? Protective or defective?

(continued)

Table 2 (continued)

- Did the subject feel threats on the childhood/parental home? Or are there any signs of overprotection?
- Are there some signs of old cracks or flaws? Had there been real misfortunes? Or imagined?
- Was there any guilt felt? Did the child attribute the burden of a fault to himself/herself? Were there any effects on self-esteem?
- What changes took place during adolescence (choices, love, desire or not to leave the parental home...)?
- What degree of fidelity does the subject feel for the parental home and the associated Ideal? Was he/she considering another Home for himself/herself? Was there any obstacle before the traumatic event? Has it changed since that event?

How is the therapist's inner world affected?
- What are the emotional movements felt by the therapist? (pity, dread, feeling of helplessness, exhaustion, anger, curiosity, excitement, etc.)
- How can the therapist's inner world reflect the client's inner world?
- What are the possible limits of empathy? (e.g. "dark areas", unspeakable painful bodily or mental experiences, gender or age or social gaps, etc.)

What objectives should be set for the reconfiguration of the inner world?
- Explore again some spatial metaphors: can the therapist glimpse "openings" of the inner world? What *horizons* can be proposed?
- How can these proposals be taken into account within the client's inner world?
- Will changes in fundamental assumptions be necessary?
- Can a unified world be found again? What are the specific obstacles to such unification?
- What are the client's untapped resources? Is there any potential for post-traumatic growth?
- Are there accessible points of support such as social models or spiritual references?
- What precautions should be taken to create a solid therapeutic framework?
- What steps and timelines can be outlined for a recovery process?
- What would be the dangers of such a process?

6   Concluding Remarks

Taking into account the client's inner world can help shape an integrative approach in PTSD, such as cognitive psychodynamics, particularly to overcome the limitations of current therapies.

Beyond the well-defined clinical framework of PTSD, such an approach can be useful in addressing traumatic situations that remain active in the subject's memory, sometimes latently, without having triggered a characterized re-experiencing syndrome in the sense of the DSM-5 or the ICD-10. Indeed, full PTSD is only the extreme of a continuum of traumatic consequences of adverse events. Such events may contribute to clinical syndromes other than PTSD, for example, adjustment disorders, complicated bereavements, but also anxiety or depressive disorders, or even somatic disorders as often observed in the elderly (Delrue & Plagnol, 2016, 2017). Moreover, unknown traumatic events can be hidden sources of intrusive interferences in working memory and influence the subject's current life (Brewin et al., 2010; Plagnol, 2004).

A detailed assessment of the coherence of the inner world can help to identify such traumatic factors, which are sometimes distant sources of the difficulties that hinder a person's fulfilment. Based on such a perspective, cognitive psychodynamics can refine the support of a person so that he or she can reintegrate into his or her inner world events that have long remained unbearable.

Points to Ponder

- If you have worked with trauma clients, to what extent have flashbacks been an important part of the presentation? Have you been able to help clients with this aspect, and if so how?
- In your experience, to what extent do clients with trauma tend to have vulnerabilities rooted in their past? How does this become evident? How would you work with this?

References

Afonso, A., Blum, A., Katz, B. F. G., Tarroux, P., Borst, G., & Denis, M. (2010). Structural properties of spatial representations in blind people: Scanning images constructed from haptic exploration or from locomotion in a 3-D audio virtual environment. *Memory & Cognition, 38*(5), 591–604.

Alim, T. N., Feder, A., Graves, R. E., Wang, Y., Weaver, J., Westphal, M., … Charney, D. S. (2008). Trauma, resilience, and recovery in a high-risk African-American population. *American Journal of Psychiatry, 165*(12), 1566–1575.

American Psychiatric Association. (2013). *Diagnostic and statistical manual of mental disorders* (5th ed.). Arlington, VA: Author.

Atwoli, L., Stein, D. J., Koenen, K. C., & McLaughlin, K. A. (2015). Epidemiology of posttraumatic stress disorder: Prevalence, correlates and consequences. *Current Opinion in Psychiatry, 28*(4), 307–311.

Baddeley, A. D. (1986). *Working memory*. Oxford: Oxford University Press.

Bremner, J. D. (2006). Traumatic stress: Effects on the brain. *Dialogues in Clinical Neuroscience, 8*(4), 445–461.

Brewin, C. R., Dalgleish, T., & Joseph, S. (1996). A dual representation theory of post-traumatic stress disorder. *Psychological Review, 103*, 670–686.

Brewin, C. R., Gregory, J. D., Lipton, M., & Burgess, N. (2010). Intrusive images in psychological disorders: Characteristics, neural mechanisms, and treatment implications. *Psychological Review, 117*, 210–232.

Briant-Davis, T., & Wong, E. C. (2013). Faith to move mountains: Religious coping, spirituality, and interpersonal trauma recovery. *American Psychologist, 68*(8), 675–684.

Bryant, R. A. (2011). Acute stress disorder as a predictor of posttraumatic stress disorder: A systematic review. *Journal of Clinical Psychiatry, 72*(2), 233–239.

Bryant, R. A., O'Donnell, M. L., Creamer, M., McFarlane, A. C., & Silove, D. (2013). A multisite analysis of the fluctuating course of posttraumatic stress disorder. *JAMA Psychiatry, 70*(8), 839–846.

Clark, A. (2013). Whatever next? Predictive brains, situated agents, and the future of cognitive science. *Behavioral and Brain Sciences, 36*, 181–253.

Conway, M. A., Singer, J. A., & Tagini, A. (2004). The self and autobiographical memory: Correspondence and coherence. *Social Cognition, 22*, 491–529.

de Lamartine, A.(1820/2001). Méditations poétiques. In A. de Lamartine, *Œuvres poétiques complètes* (pp. 1–83). Paris: Gallimard (La Pléiade).

de Lamartine, A. (1835/2001). Gethsémani, ou La mort de Julia. In A. de Lamartine, *Œuvres poétiques complètes—Voyage en Orient* (pp. 560–565). Paris: Gallimard (La Pléiade).

de Lamartine, A. (1857/2001). La Vigne et la Maison—Psalmodies de l'âme. Dialogues entre mon âme et moi. In A. de Lamartine, *Œuvres poétiques complètes, Poèmes du Cours familier de littérature* (pp. 1484–1494). Paris: Gallimard (La Pléiade).

Delrue, N., & Plagnol, A. (2016). Douleur chronique et état de stress post-traumatique chez la personne âgée. *Annales Médico-Psychologiques, 174*(5), 331–337.

Delrue, N., & Plagnol, A. (2017). Post-traumatic stress disorder in Alzheimer's disease. *Counselling Psychology Review, 32*(4), 58–69.

Fareng, M., & Plagnol, A. (2014). Dissociation et syndromes traumatiques: apports actuels de l'hypnose. *Psychiatrie, Sciences Humaines, Neurosciences, 12*(4), 29–46.

Foa, E. B., Hembree, E. A., & Rothbaum, B. O. (2007). *Prolonged exposure therapy for PTSD: Emotional processing of traumatic experiences*. New York: Oxford University Press.

Foa, E. B., Steketee, G., & Rothbaum, B. O. (1989). Behavioral/cognitive conceptualizations of post-traumatic stress disorder. *Behavior Therapy, 20*, 155–176.

Freud, S. (1915/1957). Thoughts for the times on war and death; (II) Our attitude towards death. In J. Strachey (Ed.), *The standard edition of the complete psychological works of Sigmund Freud, volume XIV (1914–1916)* (pp. 289–300). London: The Hogarth Press and the Institute of Psycho-Analysis.

Freud, S. (1915/1990). *Beyond the pleasure principle* (The Standard Edition). New York: W. W. Norton.

Freud, S. (1917/1957). Mourning and melancholia. In J. Strachey (Ed.), *The standard edition of the complete psychological works of Sigmund Freud, volume XIV (1914–1916)* (pp. 237–258). London: The Hogarth Press and the Institute of Psycho-Analysis.

Giudice, N. A., Betty, M. R., & Loomis, J. M. (2011). Functional equivalence of spatial images from touch and vision: Evidence from spatial updating in blind and sighted individuals. *Journal of Experimental Psychology: Learning, Memory, and Cognition, 37*(3), 621–634.

Grawe, K. (2007). *Neuropsychotherapy*. London: Psychology Press.

Horowitz, M. J. (1986). *Stress response syndromes* (2nd ed.). Northvale, NJ: Jason Aronson.

Horowitz, M. J. (1990). A model of mourning: Changes in schemas of self and others. *Journal of the American Psychoanalytic Association, 38*, 297–324.

Hourani, L. L., Williams, J., Forman-Hoffman, V., Lane, M. E., Weimer, B., & Bray, R. M. (2012). Influence of spirituality on depression, posttraumatic disorder, and suicidality in active duty military personnel. *Depression Research and Treatment, 2012,* 425–463.

Iacoviello, B. M., & Charney, D. S. (2016). Therapeutic adaptations of resilience: Helping patients overcome the effects of trauma and stress. In P. R. Casey & J. J. Strain (Eds.), *Trauma- and stressor-related disorders: A handbook for clinicians* (pp. 155–170). Arlington, VA: American Psychiatric Association.

Janoff-Bulman, R. (1992). *Shattered assumptions: Towards a new psychology of trauma.* New York: Free Press.

Janoff-Bulman, R., & McPherson Franz, C. (1997). The impact of trauma on meaning: From meaningless world to meaningful life. In M. J. Power & C. R. Brewin (Eds.), *The transformation of meaning in psychological therapies: Integrating theory and practice* (pp. 91–106). Hoboken, NJ: Wiley.

Johnson-Laird, P. N. (1983). *Mental models: Towards a cognitive science of language, inference, and consciousness.* Cambridge: Cambridge University Press.

Kosslyn, S. M., Thompson, W. L., & Ganis, G. (2006). *The case for mental imagery.* New York: Oxford University Press.

Lehrner, A., Pratchett, L. C., & Yehuda, R. (2016). Posttraumatic stress disorders: Epidemiology, diagnosis, and treatment. In P. R. Casey & J. J. Strain (Eds.), *Trauma- and stressor-related disorders: A handbook for clinicians* (pp. 99–118). Arlington, VA: American Psychiatric Association.

Lyon, D. R., Gunzelmann, G., & Gluck, K. A. (2008). A computational model of spatial vizualisation capacity. *Cognitive Psychology, 57,* 122–152.

Moscovitch, M., Cabeza, R., Winocur, G., & Nadel, L. (2016). Episodic memory and beyond: The hippocampus and neocortex in transformation. *Annual Review of Psychology, 67,* 105–134.

Najavits, L. M. (2015). The problem of dropout from "gold standard" PTSD therapies. *F1000Prime Reports, 7,* 43.

Plagnol, A. (1991). *Le Tragique en psychopathologie* [The tragic in psychopathology] (Medical Doctorate Thesis). University of Paris, Paris.

Plagnol, A. (2002a). L'attrition de l'espace de représentation dans les syndromes traumatiques. *Annales Médico-Psychologiques, 160,* 649–657.

Plagnol, A. (2002b). La structure pliée des espaces de représentation: théorie élémentaire. *Intellectica, 35,* 27–81.

Plagnol, A. (2004). *Espaces de représentation: Théorie élémentaire et psychopathologie* [Representational spaces: Elements and psychopathology]. Paris: Editions du CNRS.

Plagnol, A. (2014). Douleur, souffrance et intenable. *L'Evolution Psychiatrique, 79*(4), 798–808.

Plagnol, A. (in press). *Principes de navigation dans les mondes possibles* [Principles of navigation in possible worlds]. Garches, France: Terra Cotta.

Ragni, M., & Knauff, M. (2013). A theory and a computational model of spatial reasoning with preferred mental models. *Psychological Review, 120*(3), 561–588.

Resick, P. A., & Schnicke, M. K. (1993). *Cognitive processing therapy for rape victims: A treatment manual.* New York: Sage.

Samuelson, K. W. (2011). Post-traumatic stress disorder and declarative memory functioning: A review. *Dialogues in Clinical Neuroscience, 13*(3), 346–351.

Schauer, M., Neuner, F., & Elbert, T. (2011). *Narrative exposure therapy: A short-term treatment for traumatic stress disorders* (2nd ed.). Cambridge, MA: Hogrefe.

Shapiro, F. (2018). *Eye movement desensitization and reprocessing (EMDR) therapy: Basic principles, protocols, and procedures* (3rd ed.). New York: Guilford.

Shear, M. K., & Gribbin, C. E. (2016). Persistent complex bereavement disorder and its treatment. In P. R. Casey & J. J. Strain (Eds.), *Trauma- and stressor-related disorders: A handbook for clinicians* (pp. 133–154). Arlington, VA: American Psychiatric Association.

Shepard, R. N. (2008). The step to rationality: The efficacy of thought experiments in science, ethics, and free will. *Cognitive Science, 32,* 3–35.

Sherin, J. E., & Nemeroff, C. B. (2011). Post-traumatic stress disorder: The neurobiological impact of psychological trauma. *Dialogues in Clinical Neuroscience, 13*(3), 263–278.

Slater, C. L., Bordenave, J., & Boyer, B. A. (2016). Impact of spiritual and religious coping on PTSD. In C. Martin, V. Preedy, V. Patel, & B. Vinod (Eds.), *Comprehensive guide to Post-traumatic stress disorder* (pp. 147–162). Cham, Switzerland: Springer.

van der Kolk, B. (2000). Post-traumatic stress disorder and the nature of trauma. *Dialogues in Clinical Neuroscience, 2*(1), 7–22.

Ward, T., Plagnol, A., & Delrue, N. (2017). Neuropsychotherapy as an integrative framework in counselling psychology: The example of trauma. *Counselling Psychology Review, 32*(4), 18–28.

World Health Organization. (1992). *The ICD-10 classification of mental and behavioral disorders: Clinical descriptions and diagnostic guidelines.* Geneva: Author.

8

Invaded by Threat: Anxiety and Obsessive-Compulsive Thoughts

1 Introduction

Anxiety disorders can range from relatively banal phobias to major pathologies that deeply affect professional and social life. Their frequency is particularly high: anxiety disorders are the most prevalent psychiatric disorders (Bandelow & Michaelis, 2015; Bystritsky, 2006) and 33.7% of the population could be affected over the life course (Bandelow, Michaelis, & Wedekind, 2017).

Beyond the common symptom of anxiety—a sense of threat that the subject himself acknowledges as objectively unfounded—anxiety disorders are of infinite variety. These may be panic attacks, more or less frequent, or, on the contrary, a background of permanent anxiety; anxiety may be diffuse or focus on a specific type of situation; triggering events may be more external, as in phobias, or more internal, as in obsessive-compulsive disorders.

Since DSM-5 (American Psychiatric Association, 2013), obsessive-compulsive disorders are no longer included in the class of anxiety disorders, but take their place within a rather artificial class of

© The Author(s) 2019
T. Ward and A. Plagnol, *Cognitive Psychodynamics as an Integrative Framework in Counselling Psychology and Psychotherapy,*
https://doi.org/10.1007/978-3-030-25823-8_8

"obsessive-compulsive and related disorders", including, for example, trichotillomania or hoarding disorders. Such a nosographic change had been discussed all the more since the comorbidity between obsessive-compulsive disorders and phobias or panic disorders is very high (see Pallanti, Grassi, Sarrecchia, Cantisani, & Pellegrini, 2011), and pharmacological treatments are similar (Bystritsky, 2006; Marazziti, Carlini, & Dell'Osso, 2012). From our point of view, there are strong theoretical reasons for bringing together anxiety disorders and obsessive-compulsive disorders: as we will see, the cognitive-psychodynamic approach makes it possible to give a unified vision of these two types of disorders. We will therefore remain faithful to DSM-IV-TR (American Psychiatric Association, 2000) and ICD-10 (World Health Organization, 1992) by studying obsessive-compulsive disorders with anxiety disorders.

Despite considerable progress in their treatment, these disorders continue to pose clinical and therapeutic problems. Indeed, their pathogenesis remains largely enigmatic because, unlike post-traumatic stress disorder, triggering factors are far from always being found. The theoretical models struggle to explain why a particular type of symptom is observed in a given person according to his or her history. Moreover, no model clearly predicts in a unified framework the variety of these disorders, nor the existence of syndromes as specified as phobias or obsessive-compulsive disorders.

From a psychotherapeutic point of view, there are effective methods to treat most of these disorders, particularly cognitive-behavioural methods (Bandelow et al., 2017; Beck, Emery, & Greenberg, 1985; Clark & Beck, 2011; Foa, 2010; Marazitti, Carlini, & Dell'Osso, 2012; Mirabel-Sarron, Sarron, & Vera, 2018). However, it is common to observe resistance to treatment (Leahy, 2007) or that other disorders, such as depression, are revealed once the anxiety disorder has improved, sometimes associated with personality disorders that are difficult to treat (Bystristky, 2006). Some cases can be very challenging, such as the most severe obsessive-compulsive disorders, to the point that neurosurgical treatments are sometimes proposed when all chemical and psychotherapeutic methods have failed.

Taking into account the client's inner world, building on recent advances in cognitive science, it is interesting to shed light on the pathogenesis of anxiety disorders and refine their treatment by "tailoring" it to the client's needs. In this perspective, we will begin by addressing phobias, because these disorders, linked to well-defined and specific triggering situations, particularly highlight how an anxiety disorder reflects the configuration of the client's inner world. From this paradigm, we will briefly consider other anxiety and obsessive-compulsive disorders. Finally, we will specify how the cognitive-psychodynamic approach can contribute to the treatment of these disorders.

2   Phobia and the Inner World

Let's remember that a phobia is defined by the fear of being in the presence of a specified type of *external* object or situation. The subject acknowledges that his/her fear is irrational, but the encounter of such a situation triggers a panic attack and the subject does everything to avoid it, the severity of the phobia being related to the extension of avoiding.

- Agoraphobias, formerly defined by fear of open public spaces (street, square, etc.), have been extended in modern classifications (DSM-IV-TR, DSM-5, CIM-10) to fear of any situation without a way out or without accessible help or where it might be difficult or embarrassing to escape if a panic attack should occur.
- Social phobias are associated with situations that involve the presence of others, exposing the client to their "criticism".
- Many specific phobias are described: acrophobia, elevator phobia, blood phobia, animal phobia (mice, snakes, spiders, etc.), thunderstorm phobia, car driving phobia, aeroplane phobia, etc.

Sometimes a traumatic factor has a triggering role, but this is far from being the rule—for example, elevator phobias are much more frequent than actual accidents. The main models therefore highlight past predisposition situations, early adverse experiences (early life stress) with diminished (perceived) control, learning of inappropriate response, maladaptive schemas, in a context of biological/genetic or family/environment vulnerability (e.g. Beck, Emery, & Greenberg, 1985; Chorpita &

Barlow, 1998; Chorpita, Brown, & Barlow, 2016; Clark & Beck, 2011; Heim & Nemeroff, 1999, 2001; Leahy, 2002, 2007; McLeod, Wood, & Weisz, 2007; Nugent, Tyrka, Carpenter, & Price, 2011; Spence, Najman, Bor, O'callaghan, & Williams, 2002).

The behavioural approach, through progressive exposure therapies, often using virtual reality today (Botella, Fernández-Alvarez, Gillén, Garcia-Palacios, & Baños, 2017), is sufficient to cure many phobias. However, there are reluctant clients or dropouts due to fear of exposure (Leahy, 2007), and multiple and resistant phobias, associated with other anxiety or depressive disorders, against a background of personality disorders (Mirabel-Sarron, Vera, & Guelfi, 2003). In such cases, the depth and extension of the roots of the phobia in the inner world make its full recovery much more uncertain. Stagnation in treatment and "therapeutic blockages", after a brief illusion of improvement, can then be observed (Plagnol & Mirabel-Sarron, 2009).

(From Plagnol & Mirabel-Sarron, 2009)[1]

Mr K is 37 years old when he presents with a driving phobia. A senior executive, Mr K, has been married for 8 years. He and his wife are a happy couple, even if they have wanted to have a child for a long time. The problem has been going on for 10 years. Initially limited to the anxiety of passing heavyweight trucks on a highway, the phobia has spread to non-urban driving, with the anticipation of panic attacks leading to significant avoidance.

Two years earlier, treatment with antidepressants and anxiolytics relieved symptoms. Mr K maintained this treatment, without psychotherapeutic follow-up. After a promotion, confronted with an increase in his anxiety, he decided to undertake cognitive-behavioural therapy.

In addition to the phobia of driving and panic attacks, Mr K presents multiple symptoms of the agoraphobic type: phobia of public places, crowds, planes, boats, etc. There are also elements of the social phobia type, with anxiety about the look and judgement of others. In addition, Mr K has always lacked confidence in his relationships with women. Finally, a

---

[1]We are grateful to Dr Mirabel-Sarron and the review *Annales Médico-Psychologiques* for accepting that the study of Mr K's case, presented in the article cited in reference, can be widely reused here. Mr K was a client of Dr Mirabel-Sarron. Some points of this article are also mentioned in this chapter.

feeling of detachment from reality, with fear of losing oneself in a "parallel world", is sometimes pervasive. Some of these symptoms date back to adolescence, with Mr K mentioning his older sister's marriage as having triggered one of the first attacks.

Mr K is much younger than his four brothers and sisters (6 years apart from the nearest one). His father was a senior engineer and company manager, whilst his mother had devoted herself to the household. No family problems are mentioned. Mr K is surprised at his symptoms, for which he finds no "objective" reason.

Behavioural work is first proposed, with relaxation techniques and a hierarchy of exposures. The symptoms at the origin of the request decrease: Mr K can again overtake heavy trucks and regain almost complete freedom of movement, whilst the frequency of panic attacks declines significantly. His wife is expecting a child.

However, the therapist has the impression that the problems are not solved in depth. Mr K shows mentalization skills but does not seem at all ready to do without the antidepressant-anxiolytic treatment (even if it has been reduced). Relationship difficulties remain significant, related to fear of others' judgement and the induction of multiple control strategies.

To overcome a therapeutic blockage such as the one observed in Mr K, many of the cognitive therapies address the *schemas* that underlie the activation of automatic thoughts and emotions in the presence of the phobic situation (Clark & Beck, 2011; Hawke & Provencher, 2011; Leathy, 2002, 2007). In this context, schemas are metacognitive beliefs forged from past experiences that guide the interpretation of situations—for example, a recognition schema ("My life depends on the esteem of others") or a control schema ("I must control everything, otherwise...") (Leathy, 2002; Plagnol & Mirabel-Sarron, 2009). Rigid schemas can maintain phobic functioning, hence the importance of helping the subject to relax them when a therapeutic blockage occurs. However, in serious cases, the roots of such a schema can be deeply anchored in personal history and actually weigh on the entire inner world. As we will now see, it may be useful to build on advances in cognitive science, such as the representational spaces framework, to address these roots.

2.1   Phobic Core and Founding Space

When confronted with the phobic situation, the subject experiences a panic attack marked by an irrational distortion between the real situation and the catastrophic extension of the threat. The phenomenology of the crisis shows that the subject fears losing control to the point that all his ordinary space is in danger of collapsing: the part of his representational space that allows him to integrate daily events is threatened by "debacle", such as the frozen surface of a lake that breaks entirely from a localized shock (Plagnol, 2004).

Such an intense reaction to the confrontation with the phobic object, as manifested by the imaginary extension of the threat, reveals hidden tensions in the representational system that profoundly disrupt the inner world.

Sometimes, a known traumatic situation has been a real danger, with a clear associative link to the phobic situation (e.g. a car accident causing a driving phobia[2]). If this traumatic situation has not been fully symbolically worked through, it may remain a source of tension such that it is understandable that confrontation with an analogous stimulus triggers an intense emotional reaction with anxious symptoms.[3]

However, in the vast majority of cases, a traumatic factor is not detectable, especially if it is a complex phobia, combining several phobic situations and/or a panic disorder, or even other symptoms, as is the case with Mr K.

In such cases, we must admit that the phobic situation resonates through the *symbolic web* with past events and situations, recorded in memory, but not harmoniously integrated, and which remain deep sources of *conflicts* within the inner world,[4] the whole of which can be conveniently called the *phobic core*.

---

[2]For an example, see Mirabel-Sarron et al. (2018, pp. 73–74).

[3]Even if the interruption of symbolic treatment is not as premature as in the re-experiencing syndrome of the traumatic event that define PTSD (see Chapter 7).

[4]See the definitions of "symbolic web" and "conflict" in Chapter 7, Sects. 4.1 and 4.2.

Mr K (continued)

Faced with the therapeutic blockage in Mr K, a cognitive approach is proposed, with consultations being spaced 4–6 weeks apart, due to practical constraints.

Several schemas are gradually unveiled: schemas of control, judgement, vulnerability related to anticipatory fears of distress and, more in the background, a schema of recognition that seems associated with the fear of detachment from reality.

The schemas of control, judgement and vulnerability are addressed: Mr K is asked to analyse situations at the ages of 10, 20 and 30, confirming or invalidating these postulated schemas.

A different image of Mr K's family then began to emerge. The father becomes a rigid and self-centred "heavyweight"; the mother is described as devalued, always "stressed" and without a deep emotional relationship with her children. However, parental images remain relatively protected, being "excused" by the "hardness" of their children.

15 months after the beginning of cognitive therapy, whilst Mr K is working on the vulnerability schema, he recounts an episode from his childhood, around 6–8 years old, an event "forgotten" but of which he "knew full well that it would come back up". During a Sunday meal, Mr K's mother had almost choked by swallowing "the wrong way" a large piece of food and had only just been saved.

The evocation of this scene constitutes a turning point in the therapy, causing a "memory haemorrhage" and a very active investment of Mr K: he writes abundantly, reveals multiple associated memories and engages in a true inquiry in his family to reconstruct the course of events—notable differences will appear on the scenario. Mr K recovers "what he had put aside mentally", has the feeling of "opening a forgotten drawer" of his story and can recognize that his disorders are much older than what he indicated at the beginning of the therapy.

In fact, there was a heavy atmosphere in the childhood home, with paternal violence against the older siblings, whilst the mother, negated by her husband, in return adopted a passive-aggressive attitude. Against the backdrop of a threat of separation of the parental couple, everyone lived in isolation, without exchanges with the outside world (no friends, no outings, no shared entertainment, etc.). Mr K would have been protected from the father's violence by his older siblings. Since that time, only Mr K has maintained a link with all the family members who have news of each other through him.

As Mr K's case suggests, in the absence of a recent traumatic factor, the intensity of an anxiety-phobic syndrome is understandable only if the phobic situation resonates through unconscious connections with a threat to a *founding space*, i.e. an area of the representational space that gives meaning to the inner world, essential for its unification, generally associated with the construction of the ideal of the Home.[5]

The phobic core is thus formed by an ancient conflict between the founding space and the "traumatic" intuition of a possible calamity. For example, in the case of Mr K, we can assume that the phobic core is a conflict he experienced as a child between the Home and the threat of misfortune, a threat that can be symbolized by a particular scene (such as the family meal when his mother almost choked), but that is underpinned mainly by the fear of the breakdown of the family unit due to the perceived tensions in the parental couple without the child being able to understand its origin.

The encounter of the phobic situation thus acts as a probe revealing potential tensions, not apparent in day-to-day experience but deeply disrupting the inner world.

2.2   Control Space, Deviation

We now specify the logic of the development of a phobic syndrome within an inner world, as the conceptual framework of representational spaces allows us to understand it.[6]

During the formation of the phobic core, the conflict between the traumatic situation and the founding space does not break the ideal of the Home in such a way as to trigger a defence as powerful as that of a PTSD. However, the traumatic situation cannot be fully addressed and remains a source of potential tensions. Thus, in Mr K's case, the scene of maternal suffocation could have been partly symbolically worked on (it might have been different if his mother had died), but the meaning

---

[5]See Chapter 7, Sect. 4.3.2, for the definition of the Ideal of the Home.
[6]For the basis of representational spaces framework, see Chapter 7, Sect. 4.1 and Chapter 9, Sect. 2. (For a detailed theory, see Plagnol [2004, in press].)

given to it is that of a persistent threat, namely the vulnerability of the Home threatened by fragmentation.

Against the threat of misfortune, *a control space* is gradually built within the inner world to protect the founding space, with the formation of *safe zones* against the phobic core. For example, Mr K as a child was protected by his brothers, he learned to take refuge in a "safe place" (materialized by his room), and he invested in combat sports activities.

The control space can protect the subject for a long time, but the phobic core can be reactivated in later life circumstances, for example in adolescence when the departure from the parental home is on the horizon, which mentally challenges the childhood Home. K. mentions the marriage of his older sister, when he was a teenager, as the origin of the first symptoms. Later on, a professional change of course and an unfulfilled desire for a child are found as triggering factors of the phobic syndrome.

- When the phobic core is reactivated, the potential tensions it commands are actualized, but the activation is defensively deviated towards phobic zones that do not endanger the foundation space, what we will call a *deviation* process.[7] Phobic situations can thus be considered as the emerging "crests" of potential tensions on the surface of the inner world.
- The tension caused by a phobic core can be rekindled by new situations symbolically associated with it, leading to new deviations, with the gradual extension of dangerous areas, and an increase in avoidance. Each new deviation reduces the current tension, but at the same time creates a connection with the dangerous areas.
- The phobic subject must therefore increasingly monitor the "borders" of his safe zones and gradually narrow them down, especially because phobic situations attract the subject despite appearances. Indeed, the avoidance of these situations presupposes their representation and evaluation (to avoid a spider, you must activate its representation).

---

[7]In reference to Freud (1909/1955), a *displacement* can be defined as the substitution of a phobic situation for the phobic core.

Let us recall the preconscious attentional bias that phobic subjects present towards feared situations, preceding their avoidance (Mogg, Philippot, & Bradley, 2004; Rinck & Becker, 2006).

> The phobic subject therefore has no really safe shelter. The more he establishes new deviations, the more he creates paths for anguish, like a man who flees from his shadow and whose origin of fear is actually at the deep core of the Self. In major cases of avoidant personality, the subject can be compared to the inhabitant of the Kafka *Burrow* (1931/2007): each attempt to secure the burrow against the imaginary predator—e.g. by clearing an escape path—creates a new source of anxiety. The ideal of the Burrow is a safe world, but despite the appearances, the Burrow itself is full of dangers. Similarly, the phobic ideal is governed by a desire for a safe, peaceful world without dangers that could jeopardize the Home, but the Home itself conceals dreadful dangers, because of the phobic core that undermine its foundations.

2.3   Metaphor and Dimensions of Vulnerability

Taking into account, the representational space of the phobic subject has allowed us to better understand the logic of the development of a phobic syndrome in relation to the client's unique history. However, we have not yet given a real explanation for the "choice" of the phobic situation: Why do tensions in the inner world focus on a particular type of situation? Why do deviations from the phobic core lead to fear of this type of situation, in an irrational way according to the subject himself?

The inner world perspective makes it possible to address such issues, highlighting the underlying vulnerabilities to such conditions, which is important in complex phobias to avoid the risk of dropout, relapse or displacement to other symptoms.

Indeed, one working hypothesis that proves fruitful in psychotherapy is to consider that a phobic object materializes in the external space certain dimensions that make the inner world vulnerable to a traumatic agent. To put it another way, a phobic object appears as the "metaphor" for the faults in the control space (Plagnol, 2004; Plagnol & Mirabel-Sarron, 2009).

- Some dimensions of vulnerability are directly related to the structure of the inner world[8]:

  - *instability of the foundations*: the foundation space (Home) is at risk of collapse;
  - *breach*: a gap on the surface of the known world, for example a family secret, is an open door to debacle;
  - *accessibility of the centre*: the heart of the representational space—foundation space, Home, body schema, etc.—is not well protected;
  - *trap (no way out)*: there is no solution to psychic tension;
  - *dark side*: the control space and the ideal Home have a negative side.

- Other dimensions of vulnerability rather reflect the nature of the traumatic agent:

  - *power*: the agent has a high intensive energy;
  - *speed*: the agent's moves are not controllable;
  - *vitality*: the agent is alive, which makes it unpredictable (including the very important case of an agent with a mental system[9]);
  - *penetrance*: the agent has an acute/cutting profile.

For example, in aeroplane phobia, the most obvious metaphorical dimensions are those of *trap, speed* and *penetrance*. However, if we take into account the view of the Earth from an aircraft, the dimensions of *instability of the foundations* and *dark side* also play a role.

Table 1 presents the dominant metaphorical dimensions in the most common phobias. It should be noted that this dominance is relative: all dimensions of vulnerability may be present in a given phobia, but the weight of some is greater than others, which provides useful support for therapeutic work.

For example, in social phobias, the traumatic agent is the looking eyes of others: the dimension of *vitality* is all the more predominant as others

---

[8]The dimensions of vulnerability of the inner world can be rigorously defined within the conceptual framework of representational spaces (see Plagnol, 2004).

[9]The Kafka *Burrow* stops on the dreadful hypothesis of another living agent who enters the territory and turns out to be as cunning as the inhabitant whose own tricks he predicts.

Table 1 Type of phobia and dominant dimensions of vulnerability of the inner world

Phobic situation	Dimensions related to the structure of the inner world					Dimensions related to the nature of the traumatic agent			
	Instability of the foundations	Breach	Accessibility of the centre	Trap (no way out)	Dark side	Power	Speed	Vitality	Penetrance
Aeroplanes (flying phobia)	(X)			X	(X)		X		X
Thunderstorm	X	X			(X)	X	X		X
Car driving		X		X		X	X		
Small animals (mice, etc.)		X					X	X	X
Spiders			X					X	X
Elevators	X			X			X	(X)	X
Subway	X			X	X		(X)		X
Injections		X	(X)				(X)		(X)
Social situations (social phobia)								X	
Squares, markets, etc. (agoraphobia)		X	X	X				(X)	
Tunnels, caves, etc. (claustrophobia)	(X)	(X)	(X)	X	X		(X)		
Elevations (acrophobia)	X	(X)			X				
Blood (hæmophobia)		X			X				(X)

A cross between brackets indicates a less prevailing dimension are themselves subjects with their own inner worlds, leading to uncontrollable interactions; however, the eyes of others can also be associated with the idea of almost instantaneous central penetration, which involves the dimensions of *breach, accessibility of the centre, speed* and *penetration*.

The dimension of *vitality*, expressed through the eyes of others, is also important in agoraphobia, even if the most apparent dimensions of vulnerability in this type of phobia are *breach, accessibility of the centre* and *trap (no way out)*.

Let us now return to Mr K's case to show how therapeutic work can be enriched by the precise analysis of the dimensions of vulnerability of the inner world.

Mr K (continued)

After the revelation of the scene of his mother's suffocation as a child, Mr K's symptoms have disappeared, particularly in terms of relationship difficulties.

However, not everything is cloudless. Mr K does not seem to be able to do without low-dose treatment. Mr K's professional instability continues to affect him, whilst giving the impression of a certain "pleasure" of failure to achieve a more sustainable situation worthy of his skills.

In the therapeutic relationship, Mr K still gives an impression of a "smooth surface" and "screen strategies", remaining in control of the encounter. The scenario of his story is "too coherent", leaving a paradoxical feeling of confusion, as if pieces of the puzzle had not yet been put together.

The recognition schema remains present, associated with the fear of switching to a parallel world. (The film *Matrix* [Wachowski & Wachowski, 1999] is used as a metaphor.) Mr K no longer presents the phases of depersonalization that could occur during panic attacks, but a partition between several universes (and between several aspects of himself) still seems to threaten him.

This schema, which seems to be the most central, cannot be tackled directly for long, as Mr K remains in avoidance.

The work on the control and judgement schemas, in connection with Mr K's story, allowed the revelation of the scene of the maternal suffocation against the background of the "suffocating" climate of the parental home. The evocation of this scene, as it was rebuilt 30 years later, confirms several dimensions of the Home: *instability of the foundations* (threat of separation), *breach* (violent departure of the elder siblings), *trap* (isolation from the family) and *dark side* (failure of the paternal and maternal images). These dimensions, reflected throughout Mr K's inner world, are metaphorically manifested in the various phobic symptoms he presents.

However, many of the phobias presented by Mr K highlight the particular role of the *dark side* dimension, which extends beyond the Home and parental figures to reach the self-image. For example, in Mr K's phobia of driving (the initial reason for consultation), the *speed* dimension is linked to the *dark side*: Mr K actually has a masked attraction for risk-taking, like a hero who dares to defy ordinary space. In fact, Mr K sometimes engaged in risky manoeuvres on main roads, in contrast to his phobia. Similarly, the *vitality* present in the elements of social phobia reported by Mr K is associated with the *dark side* of self-image: Mr K admits to appreciating the relationship of erotic seduction that he nevertheless explicitly associates with the risk of "drowning".

This prevalence of the *dark side*, which permeates the deepest layers of Mr K's inner world—as is often the case in complex and resistant phobias—underlies the persistent weight of the recognition schema and contributes to a new therapeutic blockage. The approach of the dark side in the therapeutic setting will make it possible to overcome this blockage and open the way to even more decisive progress for a lasting recovery.

During a session in the 30th month of therapy, the problem of recognition associated with the *dark side* is confirmed: Mr K evokes the suffering in his childhood induced by his parents' indifference, as if he were "transparent" for them, otherwise it would go wrong. He remembers with emotion his successes in kung-fu competitions, congratulated by everyone, except his parents who never came to see him. For a long time, he had the feeling of being a "spectator" of the "painting" offered by a world in which he was not.

A few days after this session, Mr K carries out a project that has matured over the past six months: Mr K organizes a weekend with his four brothers and sisters, ending with a meal at his parents' house. Mr K devotes a lot of energy to bringing them together on this project, prepares the trip very carefully and shows creativity to solve the many difficulties raised by one or the other. And it is a success, leading to the first reunion in the family home since adolescence.

After the family reconciliation meal, Mr K feels that "everything is in place". He develops projects to achieve professional stability at the level he can expect. The consultations, which are held every three months, show no sign of relapse, against a background of a refined quality of exchange. From now on, Mr K only takes an anxiolytic in exceptional cases.

Admittedly, the path to recognition still seems fragile. However, Mr K now seems to accept his story in its most painful aspects and the active appropriation he shows of his life demonstrates his ability to generalize what he has discovered in the therapeutic space.

3 Generalization

We can generalize the perspective we have developed for phobias to other anxiety disorders, whether it is disorders where panic attacks occur without triggering factors related to an identified phobic situation (Panic Disorder) or those where anxiety is generalized, i.e. more diffuse over time, without "peak" acute tension (generalized anxiety disorder). Indeed, the framework of representational spaces makes it possible to model in a flexible and dynamic way, within a spatio-temporal continuum, the tensions of the inner world and their activation according to what is encountered in the outer world.

It is fruitful here to compare the inner world to an ocean traversed by areas of more or less extensive and deep zones of tension, depending on geological conditions below the surface. According to this metaphor, consciousness appears as a frail ship moving on this ocean; what appears in its window of presence is the result of interactions between what agitates the depths of the ocean and what is encountered at the surface, i.e. what comes from the outer world.[10]

---

[10]For example, the encounter of an iceberg is likely to cause a breach such that water invades the ship and eventually sinks it, despite attempts of compartmentalization, just as in post-traumatic stress disorder, as we have seen in Chapter 7, the encounter of a life-threatening experience opens a breach in ordinary space that eventually absorbs all mental life despite dissociative defences.

Building on this ocean metaphor, it is possible to develop a rigorous theory of mental navigation and its hazards.[11] However, therapeutic work can already be based on the elaboration of this metaphor with the client, and we will limit ourselves here to briefly developing it to suggest how to describe the infinite variety of anxiety disorders in the context of representational spaces.

- A panic attack reveals a zone of potential collapse of the inner world, concentrating significant tensions.[12] The subject is brutally "sucked" into the depths of his or her ordinary space, like in a maelstrom. Let's call *a vortex* the mental effects of such an internal collapse zone.
- More diffuse and less intense anxiety, without panic attacks, indicates less concentrated tensions, depending on extensive submarine reliefs, complex without being too abrupt, which orient the activation flow in an infra-conscious way. Let's call a *current* the mental effect of such a complex zone of the inner world.

Of course, all intermediaries exist between vortices and currents, just as clinically all intermediaries exist between panic attacks and generalized anxiety. In addition, vortices can coexist with currents, as well as panic attacks often occur on a generalized anxiety terrain.

- In a phobic disorder, a vortex is triggered by an encounter with the phobic situation: as we have indicated in Sect. 2.2, a phobic situation is the emerging crest of tensions in the inner world (that sometimes blossoms into a geyser). Behavioural avoidance corresponds to the setting up of safe zones, as a ship learns the passages to cross reef fields.[13]
- In a panic disorder, there is no visible crest, indicating the important role of "submarine" mental activity, i.e. interfering with consciousness, but powerful enough to form underlying vortices at the surface.

---

[11]See Plagnol (in press). We will return in Chapters 9–11 to the notion of mental navigation in a more thorough and rigorous way.

[12]Recall that the tension exerted on a (zone of) a representational space mirrors its complexity, i.e. it is inversely proportional to its degree of unification/consistency (see Chapter 7, Sect. 4.1).

[13]A traumatic factor that contributes to a phobic syndrome can be compared to the presence of a wreck that induces vortices.

Of course, crests of all sizes and intensities exist, from simple surface bubbles to giant geysers, just as clinically all intermediaries exist between panic disorders (panic attacks without triggering situation) and phobic disorders (panic attacks with triggering situations).

- In a generalized anxiety disorder, the less concentrated tensions are due to currents reflected on the surface by "swell", which can be agitated according to an infinite number of modalities, depending on encounters and atmospheric conditions ("mood"), even if activation often ends up accumulating in swirling zones, which are a source of intrusions that surge like waves to torment the consciousness (e.g. anticipation of a misfortune concerning a relative).

We hope that this marine metaphor succeeds in giving a brief overview of the richness of the theory that can be constructed within the framework of cognitive psychodynamics to account for anxiety disorders. One of the strengths of this approach is that it predicts an infinite variety of clinical forms, well beyond the "categorical" syndromes of the DSM or the CIM, which in fact offer only useful but rarely concretized benchmarks, clinical practice showing that intermediate forms or associations are much more frequent than the isolated and frank occurrence of one of these "categorical" syndromes.

Now let's show how to generalize the phobia model we proposed in the previous sections to all anxiety disorders.

- When a subject suffers from an episode of anxiety (panic attack or increase in permanent anxiety), a precise clinical analysis usually finds an external triggering circumstance, however small (e.g. a child's delay in returning from school triggers an anxiety wave on a generalized anxiety or separation anxiety terrain)[14];
- From this triggering circumstance, the subject anticipates a loss of control and/or misfortune and develops it by imagination until his/her ordinary world wavers;

---

[14]When an anxiety episode appears to be triggered by a purely internal circumstance, that is by an intrusive thought (e.g. a fantasy), clinical analysis generally finds an external circumstance that has activated the intrusive thought.

- Such an intense reaction, as manifested by the imaginative extension of the threat, reveals tensions that are not apparent in ordinary space, but deeply disturb central zones of the representational space;
- The triggering circumstance thus resonates via the symbolic web with deep sources of tension within the inner world, depending on unresolved conflicts, which are the "roots" of the disorder, or *anxious-phobic core* (generalization of the notion of phobic core introduced in Sect. 2.1). Phobic objects, torments and anxious preoccupations constitute emergences of this anxious-phobic core by unconscious connections through vortices and currents;
- The intensity of anxious-phobic syndromes, in contrast to the rational criticism of the subject, is understandable only if the defences relating to the anxious-phobic core protect a *founding space* that gives meaning to the inner world, central for its unification and associated with the Ideal of the Self (especially with the Home);
- The anxious-phobic core is thus formed by an ancient conflict between the founding space and the "traumatic" intuition of a possible misfortune, possibly driven by the subject's fantasies, if these fantasies entail a too powerful threat to the Ideal of the Self (notably to the image of the Self);
- Against the threat of misfortune, a *control space* was gradually built within the inner world to protect the founding space, with the formation of *safe zones* against the anxious-phobic core;
- When the anxious-phobic core is reactivated by a triggering circumstance, the potential tensions it controls are actualized, but the activation is defensively *deviated* towards zones that do not endanger the foundation space, which eases the tension but does not allow to go back to its source: the anxious-phobic core remains unresolved;
- When the tension linked to an anxious-phobic core is rekindled by new situations symbolically associated with it, this produces new deviations, hence the progressive extension of "dangerous" zones;
- In the absence of a phobic crest, there is no external situation that metaphorically represents the dimensions of vulnerability of the inner world (Sect. 2.3). However, it is all the more important to explore the inner world: whether or not a crest emerges, an anxiety disorder

always reveals the weaknesses of the control space and the dimensions of vulnerability of the inner world;

- In the absence of a phobic clue, systematic exploration of these dimensions of vulnerability (top line of Table 1) can be proposed to deepen therapeutic work, building on the metaphor of submarine geology, which may be associated with the Home's one[15];
- In practice, the clinician always quickly identifies dominant dimensions of vulnerability; moreover, it is rare that there is no phobia associated with panic disorder or generalized anxiety disorder, at least secondary agoraphobia, which can serve as an entry key for exploring the dimensions of vulnerability of the inner world beyond the traditional work of desensitization and cognitive restructuring.

4   Submarine Volcanoes: Obsessive-Compulsive Disorders

In anxiety disorders, triggering circumstances and internal intrusions are subject to symbolic work,[16] allowing resonances in the web of the inner world, which in principle feeds the imaginary development of a threatening anticipation from vortices or currents.

However, our theoretical framework provides for a frontier case where an internal intrusion causes major symbolic inhibition without the imaginative power being able to unfold: the intrusion causes such conflict with the consciousness that the sole symbolic work is a prohibition strong enough to remove the intrusion from the work plan without further elaboration. This is the case in an obsessive syndrome where the subject tries to cancel an obsessive intrusion by repressing or neutralizing it with compulsions.

---

[15]The two metaphors can easily be combined, for example by asking the subject to imagine a submarine palace. (Let us recall the venerable metaphors of the "mental palace" or "memory palace" associated with the famous method of loci [Legge, Madan, Ng, & Caplan, 2012; Yates, 1966].)

[16]It contrasts with the very premature inhibition of the symbolic work in post-traumatic stress disorders (see Chapter 7).

If we use our ocean metaphor again, in a pure obsessive-compulsive syndrome, the main thing happens "under the surface": the danger comes entirely from the inner world. Thus, so-called impulsive obsessions—intrusive thoughts of committing a harmful act, for example, a parent's obsession to commit aggression against his or her child, in contrast to his or her conscious feelings of pure love—reflect an ambivalence that clashes with prohibitions and is intolerable to the conscience.

However, triggering external factors are possible and all clinical intermediaries and associations exist between obsessive and anxious-phobic syndromes. For example, the worry/doubt of generalized anxiety and the scruples/doubt of "ruminating obsession" can be very similar; likewise, the "phobic obsession" of germs often associates the combination of internal intrusion and external situation (with secondary agoraphobia).

Miss J is 32 years old when she is admitted to a clinic after months of procrastination. The day before, she had slapped her young nephew with all her might because he would have inadvertently touched a knob that she herself could have touched.

She sits on the edge of the seat, avoids shaking the psychologist's hand, is concerned about her packs of self-cleaning wipes that are essential to her "survival", demands sterilized food and is worried about the laundry circuit.

Since the age of 15, she has had to perform increasingly complicated washing rituals for her hands and all body orifices, for fear of being contaminated by "germs", especially tuberculosis and sexually transmitted diseases. She says she is very informed about the epidemiology of these diseases, mentions the rampant tuberculosis and admits her "phobia" for migrants from certain Asian countries.

When she was younger, Miss J tried to resist the need to perform her rituals, conscious of their exaggeration, but the thought of contamination came back with an increasingly catastrophic magnitude: she always imagined a possibility, even a tiny one, of being contaminated herself, if only by invisible stained particles, and if she continued to resist the ritual, she would risk infecting her family and eventually the whole city—even the planet "as happened with AIDS". When her rituals are upset, she may have very violent outbursts, feared by the whole family who are enmeshed in the hell of Miss J's verifications.

> Miss J lives alone in a small apartment in the same building as her parents. She sits only on her bed and must sneak between the garbage bags arranged to collect any object she considers soiled by some contact. During rare moments of "madness", she rolls frantically in her "stained" sheets, throws everything on the floor and then empties the apartment completely; she is then calmed down for a whilst.
>
> Miss J gradually closed herself in. Around the age of 20, an affair with a young man remained platonic. After a master's thesis on Kafka, she could not continue her studies or work because she could not take public transport. In particular, she was afraid of encountering homeless people. If she goes out by exception, she throws her shoes away when she gets home and checks all her clothes for any stain. Her upbringing was both rigid and fanciful, between an austere mother and an unstable father who has spent a long time in Asia. A younger brother suffered from severe depression..

As Miss J's catastrophic fantasies about contamination show, the power of imagination is at work in obsessive disorder as well as in other anxiety disorders but encounters a power of control that is almost equal to its own.

An obsessive intrusion is immediately prohibited; however, even cancelled by the compulsion, it has existed and leaves an interfering trace, or *mental stain* (Plagnol, 2004), in the phenomenal consciousness. As with Miss J, many clinical themes of obsessive intrusion (germs, gas or water leaks, grains of sand, stained or wrinkled clothing, etc.) directly express the cruel logic of the stain.

Indeed, by clearing a stain, one risks producing a new stain. It is therefore necessary to control the clearing, then control the control, etc.—so Miss J must check that she has carried out the washing protocol correctly and complicates it even more. Each verification creates a possibility of discrepancy, therefore, a concern, a worry and an interference for the conscience, i.e. a mental stain. The obsessive subject is therefore caught in an endless spiral of control. If he/she tries to resist, the imaginative power rises, the internal tension increases until the intuition of a catastrophe, and the subject eventually gives into the ritual.

How does a subject come to lock himself/herself in behaviours from which he/she suffers so cruelly?

- The "uncontrolled" extension of the control space is only understandable if the obsessive intrusions resonate across the web of the inner world with deep sources of tension—that is unresolved conflicts—the "roots" of the disorder or *obsessive core*.
- The obsessive core here again is generally formed by an old conflict between a founding space and the "traumatic" intuition of a possible misfortune (e.g. peril on the Home). However, here the threat is also "internal" (e.g. erotic or aggressive impulses in contradiction with the Ideal of the Self and arousing guilt for endangering the Home).
- From the obsessive core, an ever-expanding control space is structured according to prohibitions. Finally, every mental path is marked out in a completely "normalized" space (Plagnol, 2004).
- The obsessive core, sometimes activated by a circumstance symbolically resonating with it, is indirectly discharged by substitutive intrusions that leave interfering stains. However, a stain-induced spiral does not allow the return to a stable normalized space.[17]
- When the subject tries to resist the rituals, a catastrophic intuition reveals the threat that endangers the depths of the inner world, that is the founding space and the Ideal of the Self, with sometimes the anguish of finding oneself without a stable Home, as Miss J. metaphorically expresses it with her fear of migrants and homeless people.
- Obsessions and compulsions reveal in a metaphorical way the form of the control space and the inner world, permeated by repressed impulses. The obsessive client is comparable to the Condemned of *The Penal Colony* (Kafka, 1919/2007): the apparently incomprehensible movement of the death machine engraves the reason for his conviction in his skin.

---

[17]Formally, it is the same problem as a water leak whose source is hidden, revealed by stains of humidity on the ceiling, stains that one would try indefinitely to erase by a paint coat, without daring to probe the walls of the home to find the source of the leak.

- The obsessive subject is thus sheared by the double scythe of his/her power of fantasy imagination and his/her almost equal power of control. Imaginative power is revealed when the normalized space "cracks", like Miss J rolling in her sheets.[18]

To use our marine metaphor once again, the obsessive world is under the influence of an underwater volcano, sometimes apparently extinguished (with coldness and conformity on the surface), but whose activity is revealed by ash emissions that mysteriously dirty the sea surface: the consciousness vainly tries to wash it, with tireless cruelty to itself, sometimes overwhelmed by the tsunami triggered by a submarine eruption.

5   Concluding Remarks

A cognitive-psychodynamic approach, grounded on the inner worlds, makes it possible to describe the very rich variety of anxiety disorders in a unified framework in which classic syndromes (phobias, generalized anxiety, obsessive-compulsive disorders, etc.) appear as boundary cases.

- The contribution of this approach can be useful especially in severe and chronic disorders that are resistant to reference therapies. Indeed, in such cases, behavioural work by progressive exposure, assuming it is possible, is often insufficient, because it remains "local" and superficial, the deep roots of the disorders being still active; likewise, cognitive work addressing schemas operates on localized problem situations that directly mobilize only small fragments of the inner world.

---

[18]Thus the Officer of *The Penal Colony* devoted himself to the absolute respect of the mechanical protocol of execution, but his fidelity to this protocol is itself a passion, and he finally throws himself into the cogs of the machine (with the words *"Be Just"* to be written on him)—which moreover horribly disrupts the machine.

- To overcome therapeutic blockages and prevent relapses, it is therefore useful to highlight with caution the roots of the disorder in the inner world. The psychodynamic cognitive approach provides a framework for gradually uncovering the deep meaning of the schemas and adjusting therapeutic objectives and methods to individual histories.
- Understanding the metaphorical value of symptoms relative to the inner world provides a powerful therapeutic lever to mobilize it. From such metaphors co-built with the client, it is often possible to highlight in a sustainable way for him dimensions of vulnerability of his/her inner world and the means to gradually overcome them, even to turn them into resources to help him to realize his/her untapped potential.
- However, the use of a therapeutic lever must be carried out at the appropriate time of the therapeutic process, i.e. as close as possible to what the client can bear, taking into account the defensive value of the symptoms and the schemas that underlie them in the inner world. It should also allow the client to access a metacognition of his/her inner world so that he can generalize the scope of the work done in therapy.

We present in Table 2 some first steps towards exploring the inner world in anxious disorders, including the exploitation of the metaphorical value of the therapeutic space itself.

The last chapters will return to the promising perspectives opened by the exploration of the inner worlds. We will see that the ability to imagine, i.e. the ability to "navigate in possible worlds", can be used in a fruitful way for the benefit of anxious clients instead of turning against them.

Points to Ponder
- In your experience, to what extent are the origins of anxiety and phobia evident in a client's history?
- How frequently do you feel that anxiety issues are rooted in a client's early development history?
- To what extent do you encourage this aspect of the client's narrative?

Table 2 First steps towards exploring the inner world in anxious disorders from the perspective of cognitive psychodynamics

---

First description of the clients' inner world
- Explore the spatial metaphors spontaneously used by the client for family and professional life ("life course", "path", "home", etc.), disease ("no way out", "darkness", etc.), therapeutic encounter ("support", etc.)
- What do these metaphors reflect about his/her inner world?
- Is it possible to use these metaphors with the client to make him/her aware of some important features of his/her own inner world?
- What precautions should be taken?
- What are the links between his/her inner world and his/her environment ("outer" world)?

Effects of the pathology on the inner world
- What are the triggering circumstances, however slight, external or internal, for anxiety symptoms?
- Are there any obsessive intrusions present? Compulsions in response?
- How to describe the incongruence between the circumstances/intrusions and the inner world?
- What are the subject's apprehensions (loss of control? misfortune?) What is the role of his/her imagination? Can he/she recognize it?
- What are the resonances between the circumstances and the inner world?
- How can the client describe the changes that the symptoms have produced in his or her inner world?
- What moves or blocking points suggest his/her emotions?
- Is there a depression? If so, what impact does it have on the inner world?
- How does the client feel about the therapeutic space between his/her inner world and the outer world? Is he/she in a "safe place"?

Resonances with the past
- What hypotheses can be made about the "roots of the disorders"? Does the client evoke it spontaneously?
- How to characterize the founding space in childhood? The Ideal of the Self? The Home?
- Did the client feel threats to the childhood/parental home? External or internal?
- Are there some signs of old cracks or flaws? Had there been real misfortunes? Or imagined? Feared?
- Was there any guilt felt? Did the child attribute the burden of a fault to himself/herself? Were there any effects of the threats on self-esteem?
- Did the subject have "safe places" and safe zones as a child? Control procedures? Rigid norms? Prohibited or taboo areas?
- What changes took place during adolescence (choices, love, desire or not to leave the parental home, etc.)?
- What degree of fidelity does the subject feel for the parental home and the associated Ideal? Is he/she considering another Home for himself/herself? What are the obstacles?

(continued)

Table 2 (continued)

How is the therapist's inner world affected?
– What are the emotional movements felt by the therapist? (boredom, anger, exhaustion, pity, positive emotions, etc.)
– How can the therapist's inner world reflect the client's inner world?
– What are the possible limits of empathy? (e.g. "dark areas", gender or age or social gaps, etc.)
What objectives should be set for the reconfiguration of the inner world?
– Explore again some spatial metaphors: what "openings" of the inner world can be glimpsed? What "horizons" can be proposed?
– How can these proposals be taken into account within the client's inner world?
– What precautions should be taken to create a solid therapeutic framework?
Are there some therapeutic levers to consider?
– Are there any blocking points? How to characterize them?
– Does the client suggest by himself/herself a metaphor that could serve as a key to addressing the vulnerability of his/her inner world?
– Are there any "phobic crests"? What dimensions of vulnerability does it suggest?
– Can the metaphor of the ocean (or the submarine palace, or the mental palace, etc.) be proposed? The metaphor of the Home? The metaphor of the volcano?
– Does the therapeutic space itself show dimensions of vulnerability? What resources does it offer? Can the identified vulnerability be transformed into a resource (e.g. *closed space/confidentiality*)?
– What metacognition of the inner world can be formed from these metaphors? How can the dimensions of vulnerability of the inner world be transformed into resources (e.g. *penetrability/exchange capacity*)?

References

American Psychiatric Association. (2000). *DSM-IV-TR: Diagnostic and statistical manual of mental disorders* (4th ed.). Washington, DC: Author.

American Psychiatric Association. (2013). *Diagnostic and statistical manual of mental disorders* (5th ed.). Arlington, VA: Author.

Bandelow, B., & Michaelis, S. (2015). Epidemiology of anxiety disorders in the 21st century. *Dialogues in Clinical Neuroscience, 17*(3), 327–335.

Bandelow, B., Michaelis, S., & Wedekind, D. (2017). Treatment of anxiety disorders. *Dialogues in Clinical Neuroscience, 19*(2), 93–107.

Beck, A. T., Emery, G., & Greenberg, R. (1985). *Anxiety disorders and phobias: A cognitive perspective.* New York: Basic Books.

Botella, C., Fernández-Alvarez, J., Gillén, V., Garcia-Palacios, A., & Baños, R. (2017). Recent progress in virtual reality exposure therapy for phobias: A systematic review. *Current Psychiatry Reports, 19*(7), 42. https://doi.org/10.1007/s11920-017-0788-4.

Bystritsky, A. (2006). Treatment-resistant anxiety disorders. *Molecular Psychiatry, 11,* 805–814.

Chorpita, B. F., & Barlow, D. H. (1998). The development of anxiety: The role of control in the early environment. *Psychological Bulletin, 124*(1), 13–21.

Chorpita, B. F., Brown, T. A., & Barlow, D. H. (2016). Perceived control as a mediator of family environment in etiological models of childhood anxiety—Republished article. *Behavior Therapy, 47*(5), 622–632.

Clark, D. A., & Beck, A. T. (2011). *Cognitive therapy of anxiety disorders: Theory and practice.* New York: Guilford.

Foa, E. B. (2010). Cognitive-behavioral therapy of obsessive-compulsive disorder. *Dialogues in Clinical Neuroscience, 12*(2), 199–207.

Freud, S. (1909/1955). Analysis of a phobia in a five-year-old boy. In J. Strachey (Ed.), *The standard edition of the complete psychological works of Sigmund Freud, Volume X (1909): Two case histories ('Little Hans' and the 'Rat Man')* (pp. 5–152). London: The Hogarth Press and the Institute of Psycho-analysis.

Hawke, L. D., & Provencher, M. D. (2011). Schema theory and schema therapy in mood and anxiety disorders: A review. *Journal of Cognitive Psychotherapy, 25*(4), 257–276.

Heim, C., & Nemeroff, C. B. (1999). The impact of early adverse experiences on brain systems involved in the pathophysiology of anxiety and affective disorders. *Biological Psychiatry, 46*(11), 1509–1522.

Heim, C., & Nemeroff, C. B. (2001). The role of childhood trauma in the neurobiology of mood and anxiety disorders: Preclinical and clinical studies. *Biological Psychiatry, 49*(12), 1023–1039.

Kafka, F. (1919/2007). In the penal colony (S. Corngold, Trans.). In S. Corngold (Ed.), *Kafka's selected stories* (pp. 35–58). New York: Norton.

Kafka, F. (1931/2007). The burrow (S. Corngold, Trans.). In S. Corngold (Ed.), *Kafka's selected stories* (pp. 162–192). New York: Norton.

Leahy, R. L. (2002). A model of emotional schemas. *Cognitive & Behavioral Practice, 9,* 177–190.

Leahy, R. L. (2007). Emotional schemas and resistance to change in anxiety disorders. *Cognitive and Behavioral Practice, 14*(1), 36–45.

Legge, E. L., Madan, C. R., Ng, E. T., & Caplan, J. B. (2012). Building a memory palace in minutes: Equivalent memory performance using virtual versus conventional environments with the method of loci. *Acta Psychologica, 141*(3), 380–390.

Marazitti, D., Carlini, M., & Dell'Osso, L. (2012). Treatment strategies of obsessive-compulsive disorder and panic disorder/agoraphobia. *Current Topics in Medicinal Chemistry, 12*(4), 238–253.

McLeod, B. D., Wood, J. J., & Weisz, J. R. (2007). Examining the association between parenting and childhood anxiety: A meta-analysis. *Clinical Psychology Review, 27*(2), 155–172.

Mirabel-Sarron, C., Sarron, P.-Y., & Vera, L. (2018). *Comment soigner une phobie avec les TCC: mieux comprendre pour mieux traiter* [How to treat a phobia with CBTs: A better understanding for a better treatment]. Malakoff, France: Dunod.

Mirabel-Sarron, C., Vera, L., & Guelfi, J. D. (2003). Psychopathologie des phobies. *Psychiatrie, Sciences Humaines, Neurosciences, 1*(1), 32–38.

Mogg, K., Philippot, P., & Bradley, B. P. (2004). Selective attention to angry faces in clinical social phobia. *Journal of Abnormal Psychology, 113*(1), 160–165.

Nugent, N. R., Tyrka, A. R., Carpenter, L. L., & Price, L. H. (2011). Gene–Environment interactions: Early life stress and risk for depressive and anxiety disorders. *Psychopharmacology (Berl), 214*(1), 175–196.

Pallanti, S., Grassi, G., Sarrecchia, E. D., Cantisani, A., & Pellegrini, M. (2011). Obsessive-compulsive disorder comorbidity: Clinical assessment and therapeutic implications. *Frontiers in Psychiatry, 2,* 70.

Plagnol, A. (2004). *Espaces de représentation: Théorie élémentaire et psychopathologie* [Representational spaces: Elements and psychopathology]. Paris: Editions du CNRS.

Plagnol, A. (in press). *Principes de navigation dans les mondes possibles* [Principles of navigation in possible worlds]. Garches, France: Terra Cotta.

Plagnol, A., & Mirabel-Sarron, C. (2009). Espace phobique et levier thérapeutique. *Annales Médico-Psychologiques, 167,* 101–109.

Rinck, M., & Becker, E. S. (2006). Spider fearful individuals attend to threat, then quickly avoid it: Evidence from eye movements. *Journal of Abnormal Psychology, 115*(2), 231–238.

Spence, S. H., Najman, J. M., Bor, W., O'callaghan, M. J., & Williams, G. M. (2002). Maternal anxiety and depression, poverty and marital relationship factors during early childhood as predictors of anxiety and depressive symptoms in adolescence. *Journal of Child Psychology and Psychiatry, 43*(4), 457–469.

Wachowski, L., & Wachowski, A. (1999). *Matrix* [Film]. Los Angeles & Burbank, CA: Warner Bros & Village Roadshow Pictures.

World Health Organization. (1992). *The ICD-10 classification of mental and behavioral disorders: Clinical descriptions and diagnostic guidelines.* Geneva: Author.

Yates, F. A. (1966). *The art of memory.* Chicago: University of Chicago Press.

9

Possible Worlds

1 Introduction

In the preceding chapters, we have highlighted some strong clinical reasons, in terms of both presenting issues and therapeutic practice, to meet in depth the inner world of the client in therapy. When we have studied depression, trauma or anxiety, to enter into the perspective from which the person sees the universe, building on the precise approach that cognitive science adopts today, was helpful to understand the roots of the difficulties and help the person to frame a way out.

In fact, as we have seen at the start (see Chapter 1), every paradigm in therapy takes into consideration the inner worlds, even if it is from an intuitive point of view. To a certain extent, therapy is nothing but the reshaping of the inner world according to a more "pleasant" perspective. For a long time, such an intuition couldn't be grounded on scientific methods. Many scholars, following Karl Jaspers (1913/1963) and his famous distinction between empathic *understanding* of others and causal *explanation*, doubted that inner worlds could ever be an object of science.

© The Author(s) 2019
T. Ward and A. Plagnol, *Cognitive Psychodynamics as an Integrative Framework in Counselling Psychology and Psychotherapy*,
https://doi.org/10.1007/978-3-030-25823-8_9

Nowadays, cognitive science offers some powerful methods to describe the inner worlds, so it becomes possible to rely on a scientific basis to understand the mental life cast by the singular story of a unique person—what has always been considered a fundamental condition of a well-founded psychotherapy. Such tools from cognitive science not only enrich cognitive behavioural therapy, but also help to integrate in a unified way the essential insights of other approaches such as psychodynamic therapy, person-centred therapy and existential therapy (see Chapter 1), so that a rich soil for a full cognitive psychodynamic approach is now ready to be fertilized, planted and harvested.

In the preceding chapters, we have only used some very limited pieces of the inner worlds. Indeed, we have only considered some fragments of the "real" world of a subject, that is, the mental representational space that constitutes the real world for this client (including the self and the therapist), with some extensions relative to his/her anticipations and desires. However, the real world or the worlds opened by anticipations and desires are only particular cases of so-called possible worlds.[1] Indeed, a human mind can embrace countless other worlds, as Walt Whitman's quotation at the beginning of this chapter strongly suggests. Fictional worlds (in novels, movies…) are obvious examples of unreal possible worlds to which we have access, but there are many other cases where a human mind seems to jump effortlessly into possible worlds: spatial travel (think of a walk in Paris or Rio de Janeiro), time travel (think of a history book that takes us into an ancient world or just remember a childhood memory), play and pretence, immersion in virtual reality, poetry reading…

In fact, possible worlds are encountered everywhere in mental life, from daily activities to high-level aspirations. Not only an alternative to the real world is involved in any anticipation, desire, fantasy, worry, entertainment (think how we slip into another world by hearing a song or viewing a movie), but possible worlds are at the heart of the most

---

[1] "Possible worlds" is a phrase whose first rigorous use is attributed to the philosopher Gottfried Wilhelm Leibnitz (1646–1716) in his metaphysical work *Theodicy* (1710/1985), but that has taken a fresh start since the work of the logician Saul Kripke who has proposed a semantic for modal logic based on "possible worlds" (Kripke, 1963).

prized activities of human beings, like erotic life (think to what flight of imagination is implied by a "love at first sight"), creativity in arts (think what is meant by "creation"), scientific enterprise (an hypothesis is nothing but the proposal of a possible state of things), metaphysical reasoning (Leibnitz was only the first in a long tradition), spiritual questioning ("Is heaven possible?")... It is so essential to the human mind to abstract from the immediate reality to explore alternatives that consciousness may rely on this ability (Baumeister & Masicampo, 2010).

To sum up, mental human life is a permanent navigation in multiple worlds, far beyond the somewhat artificial context of therapy. The inner world of a subject is a *universe* of possible worlds.

In this chapter, we will introduce new theoretical perspectives that cognitive science provides to account for the ability to navigate in the possible worlds. We have already mentioned some of them in previous chapters, but here we discuss more systematically the foundations of building a mental universe in order to have a solid basis for exploring the potential of this perspective for clinical applications in Chapters 10 and 11 (where new frontiers will be proposed for the cognitive psychodynamic approach).

After having introduced some general tools, building on striking similarities between web navigation and mental navigation (Sect. 1), we will specify some elementary conditions for a safe navigation in possible worlds, as flexible as the one we constantly practice without even being aware of it (Sect. 2).

2   A Few Basics for Mental Navigation

At first look, it could seem chimeric to define a human universe and to pretend to outline any art of mental navigation in such a universe. Philosophers are still debating about the content of elementary representations, like names, propositions or images. How can we propose to build a mental universe? The framework of representational spaces, introduced in previous chapters, will provide us with tools to take some steps to answer this question.

Let's start by noticing three daily examples of complex entities that are built from some pieces of representation:

- One very simple example is a jigsaw: by unifying the scattered pieces of a jigsaw, a coherent picture is constructed, representing a whole entity (e.g. a landscape).
- Likewise, a movie is a series of scenes that are successively "chained" on a screen to constitute a unified story.
- The Internet probably provides today the best example of a universe built from billions of limited fragments, that is millions of pages that can be displayed within a Web browser window.

These simple examples suggest that we don't need to solve hot philosophical problems about the content of the elementary representations to build a mental universe. We just need to understand *how to build complex contents from some fragments of mental presence.*

To tackle such a task, we will consider in a more detailed way the last example, the Internet, that will bring us closer to a mental system. How is the sophisticated navigation we experience on the Web possible? How does this navigation work by chaining some contents displayed in a Web browser window? In fact, it is not by chance or by some arbitrary technical choice if the Internet functions in this way. There is no other way for a representational system constrained by a limited window of presence to build a complex universe.

But perhaps a universe is a big thing. We will begin more modestly by trying to characterize what we basically do when we mentally navigate, that is when we *trace mental paths* (a very critical process for a cognitive psychodynamic approach).

2.1   Ways of Walking

Close your eyes. Think of a pedestrian path. Assume, for instance, that you are the happy Londoner Tom. You live in Kensington and you work in Mayfair. Every morning you go to work crossing Hyde Park. At every moment during your walk, a percept is displayed in your window of presence, for example, a view of Kensington Palace, a view of Albert Memorial, a view of the Serpentine, etc. All these views are "snapshots" or "scenes" that you chain in your window of presence so effortlessly that you don't even notice this chaining—it seems so naturally caused by the movement of your body!

Now, assume that you are ill. Today, you cannot get up. However, you love this morning walk so much that you decide to do it in your mind. You close your eyes and follow exactly the same route as every day—at least you try. At every moment during your walk, a mental image is displayed in your window of presence, for example, an image of Kensington Palace, an image of the Albert Memorial, an image of the Serpentine... All these images are scenes/snapshots projected from your memory that you chain in your window of presence, perhaps with a little effort if you try to be exact, perhaps effortlessly if you are satisfied with a nostalgic and somewhat fuzzy mind-wandering. You can also assume that you are a little lazy, so you are assisted by images from your computer to make the journey again. Or fond of this journey, you buy a powerful virtual reality device and you live it again in another way.

The lesson is clear. Whatever the way you make the trip, be it pedestrian, mental, combined with technical devices, or "pure" immersion in virtual reality, in all cases you must follow the same basic process: to chain some scenes/snapshots in your window of presence, exactly as when you surf on the Web you chain some pages of websites in the browser's window. In the pedestrian case, the scenes are percepts; in the mental case, the scenes are more or less vivid images projected from memory.[2] And if you do abstract reasoning, as in ethics or in mathematics, you will again chain a series of snapshots in your "mind's eye", exactly as when you do a mental walk in Hyde Park, except sensory images are replaced with more or less abstract mental models (Johnson-Laird, 1983; Plagnol, 2002, 2004, in press). There is no other way to think!

---

[2]Notice that by reading and understanding the two first paragraphs of this section you have projected a series of images from your memory. Similar mental walks are commonly used in relaxation or hypnosis.

Empirical psychology confirms that our cognitive systems operate by *scenes* (or *snapshots*, or *chunks*) integrating information over short time intervals (Nardini, Thomas, Knowland, Braddick, & Atkinson, 2009; Newman, Choi, Wynn, & Scholl, 2008; Rubin & Umanath, 2015), even if these intervals aren't perceived (as in cinema we do not feel the interval between two images for the benefit of a continuous phenomenal experience).

A scene corresponds to the content at a given moment of the *spatial array* of the working memory,[3] which can receive sensory inputs as well as image projections from long-term memory.[4]

Perceptions and mental images are *depictic* (or *analogical*, *pictorial*, *iconic...*) in the sense that they immediately present some contents. According to *grounded cognition* (Barsalou, 1999, 2008), any representation is based on depictic components. Conceptual frameworks such as *mental models* (Johnson-Laird, 1983), *embodied cognition* (Glenberg, 1997), *perceptuals symbols* (Barsalou, 1999), show how to build the representation of abstract entities from depictic components, i.e. from scenes that can be deployed within the spatial array of working memory.

2.2   Web Navigation and Mental Navigation

In the first era of cognitive science, in the 1950s, and until the 1980s, the comparison between human minds and computers was very popular. However, advances in cognitive science have highlighted the limitations of such a comparison—for example, the inability of a computer to flexibly adapt to a changing environment. Contrary to classical computers, animal organisms are remarkably able to adapt to their environment, so cognitive science has taken a recent inspiration from the Theory of Evolution (e.g. Platek & Shackelford, 2009). However, a

---

[3]See Chapters 2 and 8. We define more rigorously the "window of presence" in Sect. 2.3 below.

[4]Perceptions and images are deployed within the spatial array in similar ways and elicit the same type of treatment (Borst & Kosslyn, 2008; Ciaramelli, Rosenbaum, Solcz, Levine, & Moscovitch, 2010). Mental imagery uses structures developed for perception (Ganis, Thompson, & Kosslyn, 2004; Kosslyn, 1994), whilst any perception is largely projective (Clark, 2013; Soto, Wriglesworth, Bahrami-Balani, & Humphreys, 2010).

much stronger model can be found in a system that we daily use today: as soon as we take the point of view of the represented universe, we understand that the World Wide Web can provide very useful tools to describe a mental universe.[5]

- At first, the mental representation of any object can be compared to a website. Indeed, such a representation in a mental space is nothing but a collection of scenes/snapshots/chunks that are integrated together thanks to a unit key, that is a symbol (a mental name), exactly as a website is a collection of pages that are unified by a Web address.[6] For example, your favourite park in your mental space is a collection of mental images connected by a mental name like *Hyde Park*. More abstract objects, like moral or mathematical objects, have the same type of structure, except that sensory images are replaced with mental models. Indeed, all the mental objects are structured in the same way, exactly as all the websites are structured in the same way independently of the nature of their contents.
- If the mental name of an object O is activated, it acts as a retrieval cue to recall in the window of presence some snapshots of O, exactly as a Web address allows access to the pages of a website. For example, if *Hyde Park* is activated in your memory, it acts as a retrieval cue and may give rise to the projection of a mental image of Hyde Park in your window of presence.[7]
- From mental objects, we build more complex fields, thanks to links between their names, that is, thanks to a network of symbols (or *web*), just like connecting some websites by hypertext links to build

---

[5]Reciprocally, building a model of the inner world displayed by a representational system can draw a new light on the current limits of artificial intelligence.

[6]Likewise, a visual object is nothing more than an *object file* identified by a pointer or index "tracking" the identity of a "target" through changes in place and properties (Feldman & Tremoulet, 2006; Kahneman, Treisman, & Gibbs, 1992; Mitroff, Scholl, & Wynn, 2005).

[7]However, unlike a website, a mental object is essentially dynamic. The memory processes of coding allow to decompose a scene/snapshot and to recombine the pieces into new fragments according to the active memory context (see Plagnol, 2002, 2004, in press). You may have stored in memory only a few percepts about Hyde Park, but it is sufficient to give rise to a potential infinity of mental images of Hyde Park in your window of presence.

more sophisticated networks on the Internet. For example, the development of autobiographical memory can be considered as the progressive formation of a "glue" that unifies the first scattered pieces of memory (Bauer, 2015), in parallel with the development of verbal/symbolic representations, until a coherent narrative emerges, so at maturation, generally not before 8–9 years, an individual begins to be able to navigate in his/her own story.

- Finally, the totality of our mental fields form a rich and ever-changing mental universe in which we are able to trace an infinity of mental paths, even if we only actualize a very tiny fraction of them during our life, as we only explore a very tiny fraction of the billions of Web pages.

A rigorous construction of a mental universe is possible (see Plagnol, 2004, in press), but the underlying intuitions are very simple and we don't need here to bother with cumbersome tools to address the basics of mental navigation. Indeed, everybody understands by experience what it means to "navigate the Web"; the parallel with the navigation in a material space is straightforward, and navigation within a mental space depends basically on the same processes. From a formal cognitive point of view, there is no significant difference between following a path on the Internet, following a path in a material space, and following a path in a mental space: in all cases, it comes down to chaining some scenes/snapshots in a window of presence.

2.3   A Few Definitions

Let's take the time to build up a stock of some clear-cut definitions. It may look a bit formal, but it will allow us to base on firm ground the intuitive ideas we have introduced, so that we can explore the inner worlds in a sufficiently rigorous way to meet the ambitions of the cognitive psychodynamic approach.[8]

---

[8]Some of these ideas have been introduced in the previous chapters.

Assume a mental system MS. To fix the ideas, we will consider that MS is the mental system of the Londoner Tom. (Think of your own mental system if you prefer.) We start with the fundamental notion of window of presence already mentioned in this chapter as well as in Chapters 2 and 7.

- The window of presence *of MS* is the capacity of maximal co-display of the MS. In contemporary psychology, the window of presence is implemented as a *work space* (Baars, 1994) whose main displayed content corresponds to the working memory's "visuo-spatial" component (Baddeley, 1986)—or *work plan* (Plagnol, 2002, 2004, in press), *spatial array* (Ragni & Knauff, 2013), *spatial field* (Lyon, Gunzelmann, & Gluck, 2008).[9] The usual human window of presence is bounded, has a finite power of resolution, has no more than three dimensions and is constrained by a Euclidean geometry.[10]
- An *elementary fragment* for MS is a representational fragment that can be displayed in the window of presence of MS.[11] A *situation* is the immediate content of an elementary fragment. Percepts, mental images or mental models are elementary fragments that present more or less abstract situations. For example, a percept of the Serpentine in Hyde Park directly displays a sensory aspect of the Serpentine (say, a bit of a watercourse bordered by some grass); a more abstract mental model of the Serpentine may display a blue schematic ribbon that undulates amongst green spots.

---

[9]See Chapters 2 and 7. Recall that what is important is the spatial display at a given time, not the usual sensory modality underlying this display, and that *work plan* emphasizes that the displayed content is subject to mental processing (i.e. why we use this term in the following).

[10]Here we only consider mental representations that are able to enter the conscious flow of the phenomenal experience. Constraints can be different for other cognitive levels.

[11]In Chapter 7, the elementary fragments were called "*analogical* fragments" because Chapter 7 focused on their *depictic* format, which is in contrast to that of *symbolic* representations. Here, we focus instead on the *elementary* character of these presence fragments from which complex entities are constructed. As mentioned above, the grounded cognition framework (Barsalou, 1999, 2008) offers strong reasons to admit that elementary fragments of representation are analogical (or depictic, iconic…).

A situation cannot exceed the limits of the window of presence. Thus, in order to reconstitute extended contents, elementary fragments need to be chained and successively displayed within the window of presence; moreover, the fragments that aren't displayed at a given instant in the window of presence must be coded and stored within a memory (as the pages of a website are coded and stored on a server). A network of symbols can enact these different functions (as already mentioned in Chapter 7, Sect. 4.1).

- The *symbolic system* (or *web*) of a representational system is the system of entities (*symbols*) that is used to code the elementary fragments, store these fragments in their coded format and chain the reactivated fragments in the window of presence.

The symbolic system yields access to contents that are larger, more precise and more complex than the situations directly displayed by the analogical fragments. As there are links between symbols, each symbol can be considered as a *node* of the web. Each node is more or less activated at a given time.

- An *extension* for MS is the unification of several situations thanks to the web of MS.

An extension E cannot wholly immediately be present in MS if it exceeds the window of presence of MS, but E can be *virtually* available by MS, in that it is possible to *navigate* within E thanks to MS, by chaining successive elementary fragments in the window of presence.

For instance, each mental image of London that Tom is able to project into his window of presence from his memory is an elementary fragment for his mental system; the unified set of these mental images forms a virtual model of London within which Tom may navigate, even though Tom is unable to wholly display this model at a given instant.

- A *mental object* O is an extension organized around a characteristic symbolic unit (or *name*)—that is, a specific coding unit that connects the different representational fragments that constitute O. For example, the elementary fragments of Tom relative to London are organized around his mental name *London*.

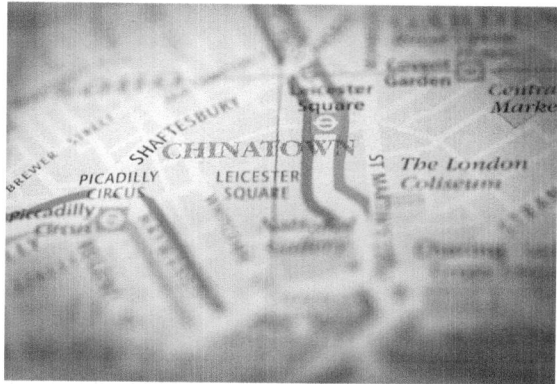

Fig. 1 Making a mental journey across London

- A *path* from a situation S to a situation S' is a series (S,..., S') of situations that can be successively displayed in the window of presence.
- A *symbolic structure* is a web fragment that allows a path to be constructed.[12]

For example, during a daydream about London, Tom can follow a mental path from Covent Garden to Piccadilly Circus through Leicester Square thanks to a series of images that are successively projected in the spatial array of his working memory and chained by a symbolic structure using links between his mental names *Covent Garden, Leicester Square* and *Piccadilly Circus* (Fig. 1).

- The *universe* U represented by Tom is the union of all extensions of MS.

Tom can mentally navigate in this universe by charting paths. An infinity of situations can be projected from his long-term memory (that stores millions of mental objects),[13] so U conceals an infinity of paths, all the more as new fragments are continually added by perception and

---

[12]A symbolic structure is the mental equivalent of a series of hypertext links on the World Wide Web.

[13]See Note 8 of this chapter.

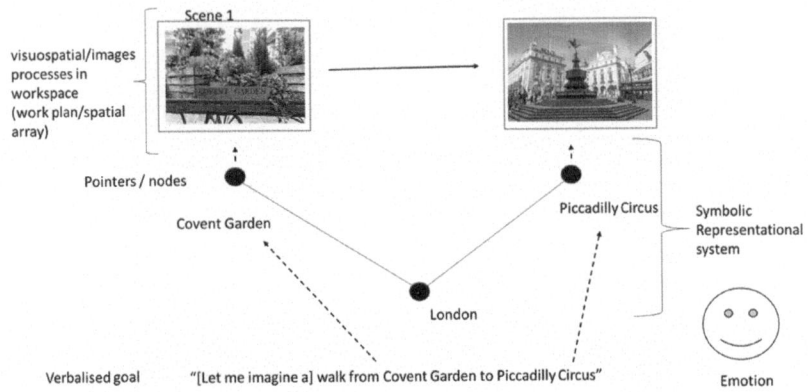

Fig. 2 The global workspace processes involved in making a mental journey across London

other mental activities. An illustration of these processes is given in Fig. 2. In the figure, Tom verbalizes his current goal as to "imagine a walk from Covent Garden to Piccadilly Circus", and each of these place names activates the relevant pointer/node. These nodes then link to and activate the relevant visual fragments with the visuospatial processes. The smiley face is simply to make the point that the global workspace can include many different types of representation, including feelings. In this case, we assume that Tom enjoys his walk through London, and imagining it recreates a sense of happiness.

3   Requirements for a Safe Navigation

We can evolve at high speed in complex universes of multiple worlds whilst at a given moment only a few tiny fragments of world are displayed in our presence window. In particular, we do not generally mix worlds that are considered different. In this section, we will specify the basic constraints that must be met for such navigation, and then show that a functional partitioning mechanism between mental representations is sufficient to meet these requirements in an effective and flexible way.

3.1   An Amazing and Early Ability

Every parent reads stories to his/her children at night to put them to sleep. Each story defines a different world and the child does not mix these worlds—if necessary he/she reminds tired parents that this character is in one story and not another! From the age of five, children are able to manage complex interlocking worlds.

For example, in *Peter Pan* (Barrie, 1911/2004), the world of Neverland is nested in the fictional world, itself nested in the real world. In addition, the child must represent the "replicas" of characters from one world to another, as is the case for Wendy and her brothers in *Peter Pan*—Wendy even encounters some characters she has invented!

In other stories, some characters dream, which implies representing the world of the dream nested in the fictional word. The distinction may even become clear only at the end of the story, like in *Alice's adventures in Wonderland* (Carroll, 1865/2009), but no problem, the child understands this ultimate rebound, which means that he/she can almost instantly update his/her representation of the different worlds in the correct way. The child can also switch into past worlds (e.g. by reading a story about William the Conqueror), or mix past worlds with fiction (e.g. by reading a story about [the legendary] Robin Hood), or slip into (fictional) future worlds (by reading a science fiction novel). Lastly, he/she can enter into worlds represented by characters, for example, to understand their motivations and tricks.

Think of the famous episode of the poisoned apple in *Little Snow White* (Grimm & Grimm, 1812/2011). It seems to be a relatively simple trick. However, to understand it, the child must represent the inner world of the witch (*alias* the evil queen) and the inner world of Snow White, with the difference of these two worlds concerning the apple and the identity of the old woman (*alias* the witch, *alias* the evil queen) who offers the apple. In representing the inner world of the witch, the child must represent how the witch represents herself in the inner world of Snow White (who doesn't know that the apple is poisoned) and how the witch

> represents to herself a desired scenario (the death of Snow White after eating the apple)—*desired*, therefore not yet real and to be distinguished from the present reality of the tale, itself of course distinguished from the current real world of the child.

As adults, we also constantly use multiple, heterogeneous and nested worlds, with numerous replicas of characters.

> Think of a literature student, Sally, who studies a commentary on Homer's *Odyssey* by the scholar Victor Bérard. Sally can easily represent that Bérard thought that in the mythology of Homer, Ulysses admitted that Penelope thought that the Suitors imagined that Ulysses had no idea what was going on in his palace. In terms of possible worlds, Sally represents the world of Bérard representing the world of Homer representing the world of mythology in which Ulysses represents the world of Penelope representing the world of the Suitors representing what Ulysses represents what is happening in his palace—a very contrived wording, whilst Sally reads smoothly the Bérard's commentary!

As the above examples suggest, without even being aware of our achievements, we can easily manage:

a. different worlds without confusing them or confusing them with the real world;
b. nested worlds on several levels and move between them;
c. entangled worlds of different types (fictional, mental/epistemic, temporal...);
d. replicas (or *avatars* or *counterparts*) of the same individual from one world to another; and
e. orientation in different worlds to know almost instantly in which we are in, in particular relative to the real world (like in the end of *Alice's adventures in Wonderland*).

(a)–(e) define the minimum constraints that a cognitive system must meet to navigate in the possible worlds and we will specify below how a mental system succeeds at this. However, before we tackle this task, we must add some important qualifications.

3.2   Caveats

Even if we have insisted on our mental ability to navigate between different worlds, there are many reasons why we can confuse different worlds:

- We have put forward the navigational exploits a child is capable of, but a certain maturity of the mental system is necessary to master the management of several worlds. A three-year-old child is capable of pretend play (Friedman, Neary, Burnstein, & Leslie, 2010), can differentiate the real/imaginary status of characters (Corriveau, Kim, Schwalen, & Harris, 2009), or distinguish the world of others from his or her own (Buttelmann, Carpenter, & Tomasello, 2009), but separation between different worlds may be difficult to maintain at this age due to limitations in working memory (Scott, Baillargeon, Song, & Leslie, 2010).
- We have already mentioned the case of the tired parent when reading a story at night. This situation is a particular case of conditions in which the functional state of memory can induce confusion between worlds. In many physiological, emotional or pathological states, we can mix worlds inappropriately. For example, in a dissociative state (mythomania, state of trance, deep reverie…), we typically merge an imaginary world with the real world. Or if we take a drug like LSD, we quickly blur the boundaries between worlds, starting with the boundary between imagination and reality. A small alcohol intake can accelerate our thinking speed so that fantasies and reality merge. Let's also remember that a psychotic person tends to mix the therapist's world with his/her own world.
- Because of changes in our mental space over time, we can confuse worlds that we have first been able to distinguish, notably because of the weakening of encoding contexts and interference between sources of information (Ecker, Lewandowsky, & Tang, 2010; Goff & Roediger, 1998; Hyman & Pentland, 1996). For example, we can mix *Richard II* and *Richard III* of Shakespeare (whom we knew by heart in our youth), confuse *River of no return* (Preminger, 1954)

and *Rio Bravo* (Hawks, 1959) having watched both a hundred times, attribute a passion for strawberries to our fiancée Sally instead of attributing it to our former girlfriend Suzan, take King's Cross Station in 2017 for Kings' Cross Station in 1993.... We may even end up considering false memories or imaginary events as real (McDonough & Gallo, 2010; Nash, Wade, & Lindsay, 2009; Zaragoza, Mitchell, Payment, & Drivdahl, 2011).

Thus, many structural or functional conditions of memory can lead to confusion between worlds. Conversely, a world in principle unified can be mentally fragmented. For example, although the representations associated with the *Iliad* and the *Odyssey* are in principle unifiable into one Homeric World, a reader may sometimes consider them to involve two distinct worlds.

3.3   Functional Compartmentalization

The adequate mental representation of possible worlds must allow:

1. the distinctions between different worlds;
2. the unification of elements belonging to the same world; and
3. inappropriate fusions or fragmentations under certain conditions.

Such requirements can be easily ensured in a mental space by a functional process of *compartmentalization* (Plagnol, 1993, 2004, in press; Plagnol, Pachoud, Claudel, & Granger,1996; Potts & Peterson, 1985; Potts, St. John, & Kirson, 1989):

- Recall that a mental object is associated to a specific cue, a mental name, which is also a node in the web and a retrieval cue for the different aspects of the object. Now, from a cognitive point of view, a mental world is only a special case of object, and a name is associated to each mental world.
- For example, each novel you read defines a specific world and the title of the novel offers a natural name to this world, associated to all the objects and events of this world. If your mental key *Peter Pan*

is activated—e.g. by reading "Peter Pan"—you can recall the world of *Peter Pan* (Barrie, 1911/2004), and the different events in this fictional world, because all your items relative to this world in your memory are connected to the node *Peter Pan* in your mental web. If your six-year-old daughter says "Wendy is brave", you will find the right Wendy if you remind yourself that you have recently read *Peter Pan* with your daughter and you reactivate the Wendy of *Peter Pan* thanks to the link in your mental web between a node *Wendy* and the node *Peter Pan*—so you do not confuse the *Peter Pan*'s Wendy with the neighbour's wife who is also called Wendy.

- A *compartment* is an isolable memory zone thanks to a web node (name) specifically connected to all the elements composing this zone. Let it be a world W in a mental universe U, to which corresponds a node N(W) in the web of U: if all nodes encoding content belonging to W are associated by powerful links to N(W), N(W) defines a compartment for the world W.

Compartmentalization can ensure the structuring of a mental universe into distinct worlds (so the constraint [a] above is fulfilled). However, such a structuring is functional and can be blurred under certain conditions. If the links to the world nodes are relatively weak, for example, because the available activation is attracted elsewhere, compartmentalization is no longer ensured and distinct worlds may tend to merge.

Figures 3 and 4 represent the results of an experiment on the understanding of fictional stories by non-clinical participants and people diagnosed with schizophrenia (Plagnol, 1993; Plagnol et al., 1996). Each participant had to read a series of six texts telling six brief fictional stories. After reading, the proximity of the representations in memory was studied by a word recognition technique with priming. In the non-clinical population (Fig. 3), the results show that two words from the same story are closer in memory than two words for different stories. To give a detailed account of all the results, it is necessary to postulate a world node for each story to which all the items related to this story are strongly connected. In people with schizophrenia (Fig. 4), everything happens as if the connections allowing compartmentalization were blurred because of interfering sources of activation (which can be related, for example, to hallucinatory voices).

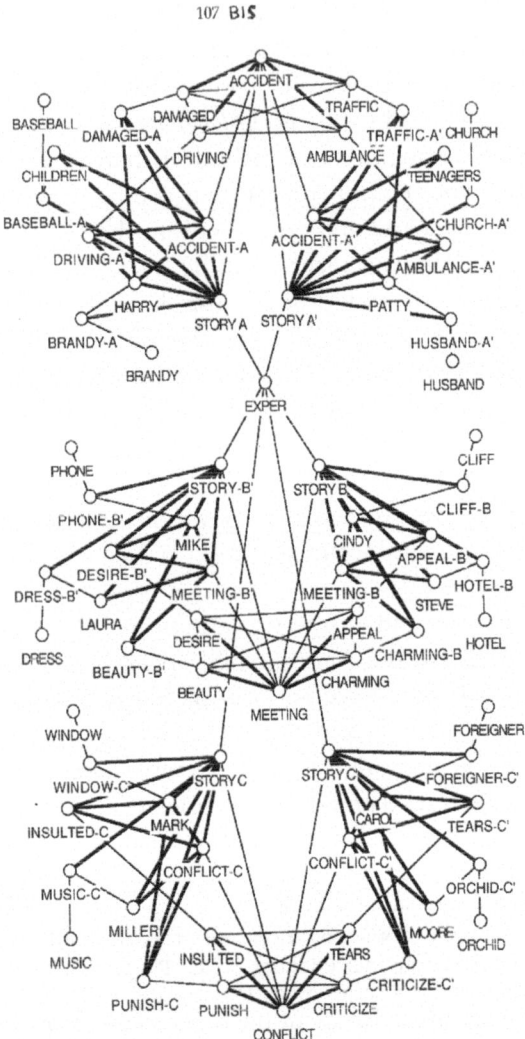

Fig. 3 Representation of fictional narratives by non-clinical subjects (From Plagnol, 1993, p. 107bis. The worlds nodes are the nodes "Story A", "Story A'"... The thicker a link is, the more powerful it is. See the six compartments on the figure [each is controlled by a story node]. The six stories were also paired by thematic topics that correspond to other contextual nodes ["ACCIDENT", "MEETING", "CONFLICT"]. The node "EXPER" represents the experimental context)

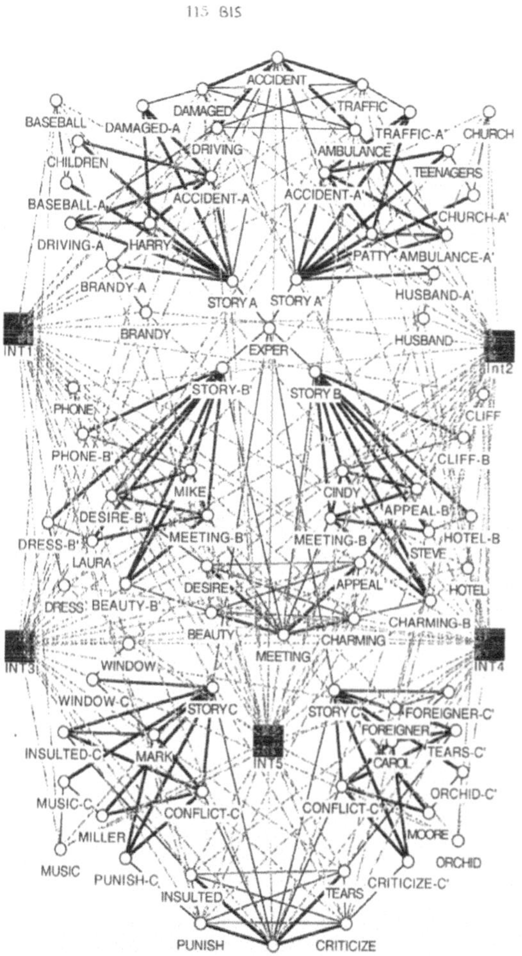

115 BIS

Fig. 4 Representation of fictional texts by people with Schizophrenia (From Plagnol, 1993, p. 115bis. Compared to Fig. 3, the six-compartment structure is blurred. The hypothesis of powerful interfering activation sources [INT1 to INT5 nodes] accounts for this

Let's highlight four points that show the efficiency and flexibility of such a functional compartmentalization process:

1. The notion of compartment is not specific to possible worlds. Memory areas can be functionally isolated without corresponding to a possible world. Indeed, any marked context defines a functional compartment. Activation networks such as those deployed in Figs. 3 and 4 allow the flexible and dynamic implementation of any type of compartment. For example, the EXPER node on these figures represents the context of the experiment. In fact, the compartmentalization of possible worlds offers a paradigm for studying the contextualizing effects that are so important in information processing, especially in conditions such as schizophrenia.[14]

2. World nodes that ensure compartmentalization can be considered as *pointers* (or *tags*). Their functional assignment to an item is sufficient to mark this item as belonging to this or that world, whatever the type of world concerned: fictional, temporal, mental/epistemic… So functional compartmentalization is efficient to represent entangled worlds (see the constraint [c] set out in Sect. 3.1). Moreover, the links between pointers can be "vertical" and ensure nesting between worlds (see the constraint [b] in Sect. 3.1).[15]

3. The compartmentalization by a set of pointers is also very economical: the construction of a possible world is limited to what differentiates it from the reference world and is marked by its specific world pointer/node. No need to reconstruct an entire world: only facts specific to that world are represented and tagged. Similarly, a replica of an entity in a possible world is simply defined by what differentiates it from the replica in the reference world (see constraint [d] in Sect. 3.1). *Peter Pan*'s Wendy is the same in the initial world at the beginning of the story and in Neverland, except that the adventures that

---

[14]Functional decontextualization of representations is at the heart of cognitive troubles in schizophrenia (see Plagnol et al., 1996).

[15]More generally, such vertical links can functionally represent nesting contexts (Plagnol, 1993, in press). For instance, within Figs. 3 and 4, the six fictional story nodes depend on the node EXPER that represents the experimental context.

happen to her in Neverland are specific to this world and are marked as such.

4. The state of activation of the pointers makes it possible to locate oneself between the worlds (see constraint [e] in Sect. 3.1) and to navigate between them. It is sufficient that the world in which we are located is indicated by the most active pointer in our presence window, just as the brighter tab on the window of a browser on the Internet can make it possible to know on which web site we are located.

Pointer activity adjustments allow us to move very quickly from one world to another, as when one reactivates a Web browser window to bring it to the foreground by clicking on the tab that controls it. For example, when we read *Peter Pan*, we can immerse ourselves into Neverland, but in principle we keep an active *Neverland* pointer in our presence window that lets us know we are in Neverland (and not in the real world or in some other fictional world). Notice that this *Neverland* pointer is itself linked to the *Peter Pan* pointer, active in the background: when at the end of the story, Wendy leaves Neverland to return to *Peter Pan*'s basic world, we reactivate our *Peter Pan* mental node and deactivate our *Neverland* node. And if we really want to leave this wonderful story, we "click" on (our) real world—the default world, therefore the only one that doesn't need a specific tag—and deactivate our *Peter Pan* node.

> When we wake up from an intense dream, we switch in principle to the reference window (by default the real world as perceived), but the dream window is sometimes still strongly active, and we can have a moment of floating between what is dreamlike and what is real. Perceptual cues such as a wake-up bell usually serve as strong pointers to reality and we quickly encapsulate/compartmentalize the elements of the dream with an appropriate pointer. Likewise, when Alice wakes up at the end of her dream to return to the basic world of *Alice's adventures in Wonderland*, the unfamiliar reader may have a moment of floating, but he/she quickly encapsulates the elements of Wonderland by marking them with a world node *dream of Alice* and only has to add a vertical link between that node and his/her *Alice's adventures in Wonderland* node.

4   Concluding Remarks

Cognitive science provides today powerful concepts to account for our outstanding ability to navigate through possible worlds. Such an ability being involved in all the dimensions of mental life, its study is necessary to fully capture the richness of a human universe and ground a cognitive psychodynamic approach that fulfils all its promises.

Internet navigation offers an inspiring model for exploring the inner worlds. However, our mental system works in a much more flexible way than the World Wide Web, because the mental compartmentalization is functional—whereas the organization of the sites on the Web is finally rather rigid—and is constantly changing according to the activation levels of the nodes of the mental frame.

In particular, we are able to very quickly modulate the degree of compartmentalization of a world W relative to other worlds, depending on the intensity of the immersive experience we need in W. For example, we can immerse ourselves deeply in the world of a play like *Hamlet*, then leave it to take an interest in the theatre stage and the actor's acting—the pleasure aroused by such a back and forth between real and fictional world is essential to the tragic spectacle as Aristotle already pointed out in *Poetics* (335BC/1996).[16]

In general, such flexibility in structuring possible worlds allows for an infinite variety of emotions in "mental navigation", as can be exploited in poetry, literature or music, but also in therapy, as we will see in the following chapters.

References

Aristotle. (335BC/1996). *Poetics* (M. Heath, Trans.). London: Penguin Classics.

Baars, B. J. (1994). A global workspace theory of conscious experience. In A. Revonsuo & M. Kamppinen (Eds.), *Consciousness in philosophy and cognitive*

---

[16]It can also easily be observed in an infant during a pretence game (Leslie, 1987).

neuroscience (pp. 149–171). Hillsdale, NJ: Lawrence Erlbaum Associates, Inc.

Baddeley, A. D. (1986). *Working memory.* Oxford: Oxford University Press.

Barrie, J. M. (1911/2004). *Peter Pan.* New York: The Modern Library.

Barsalou, L. W. (1999). Perceptual symbol systems. *Behavioral and Brain Sciences, 22,* 577–660.

Barsalou, L. W. (2008). Grounded cognition. *Annual Review of Psychology, 59,* 617–645.

Bauer, P. J. (2015). A complementary process account of the development of childhood amnesia and a personal past. *Psychological Review, 122*(2), 204–231.

Baumeister, R. F., & Masicampo, E. J. (2010). Conscious thought is for facilitating social and cultural interactions: How mental simulations serve the animal-culture interface. *Psychological Review, 117*(3), 945–971.

Borst, G., & Kosslyn, S. M. (2008). Visual mental imagery and visual perception: Structural equivalence revealed by scanning processes. *Memory & Cognition, 36*(4), 849–862.

Buttelmann, D., Carpenter, M., & Tomasello, M. (2009). Eighteen-month-old infants show false belief understanding in an active helping paradigm. *Cognition, 112,* 337–342.

Carroll, L. (1865/2009). Alice's adventures in Wonderland. In L. Carroll (Ed.), *Alice's adventures in Wonderland & through the looking glass* (pp. 9–128). London: Macmillan.

Ciaramelli, E., Rosenbaum, R. S., Solcz, S., Levine, B., & Moscovitch, M. (2010). Mental time travel in space: Damage to posterior parietal cortex prevents egocentric navigation and reexperiencing of remote spatial memories. *Journal of Experimental Psychology: Learning, Memory, and Cognition, 36*(3), 619–634.

Clark, A. (2013). Whatever next? Predictive brains, situated agents, and the future of cognitive science. *Behavioral and Brain Sciences, 36,* 181–253.

Corriveau, K. H., Kim, A. L., Schwalen, C. E., & Harris, P. L. (2009). Abraham Lincoln and Harry Potter: Children's differentiation between historical and fantasy characters. *Cognition, 113,* 213–225.

Ecker, U. K. H., Lewandowsky, S., & Tang, D. T. W. (2010). Explicit warnings reduce but do not eliminate the continued influence of misinformation. *Memory & Cognition, 38*(8), 1087–1100.

Feldman, J., & Tremoulet, P. D. (2006). Individuation of visual objects over time. *Cognition, 99,* 131–165.

Friedman, O., Neary, K. R., Burnstein, C. L., & Leslie, A. M. (2010). Is young children's recognition of pretense metarepresentational or merely behavioral? Evidence from 2- and 3-year-olds' understanding of pretend sounds and speech. *Cognition, 115,* 314–319.

Ganis, G., Thompson, W. L., & Kosslyn, S. M. (2004). Brain areas underlying visual imagery and visual perception: An fMRI study. *Cognitive Brain Research, 20,* 226–241.

Glenberg, A. M. (1997). What memory is for. *Behavioral and Brain Sciences, 20,* 1–55.

Goff, L. M., & Roediger, H. L., III. (1998). Imagination inflation for action events: Repeated imaginings lead to illusory recollections. *Memory & Cognition, 26,* 20–33.

Grimm, J., & Grimm, W. (1812/2011). Little snow white. In The Brothers Grimm (Eds.), *Grimm's complete fairy tales* (pp. 187–194). San Diego, CA: Canterbury Classics.

Hawks, H. (1959). *Rio Bravo.* Burbank, CA: Warner Bros.

Hyman, I. E., Jr., & Pentland, J. (1996). The role of mental imagery in the creation of false childhood memories. *Journal of Memory and Language, 35,* 101–117.

Jaspers, K. (1913/1963). *General psychopathology* (J. Hoenig & M. W. Hamilton, Trans.). Chicago: University Chicago Press.

Johnson-Laird, P. N. (1983). *Mental models: Towards a cognitive science of language, inference, and consciousness.* Cambridge: Cambridge University Press.

Kahneman, D., Treisman, A., & Gibbs, B. J. (1992). The reviewing of object files: Object-specific integration of information. *Cognitive Psychology, 24,* 175–219.

Kosslyn, S. M. (1994). *Image and brain: The resolution of the imagery debate.* Cambridge, MA: MIT Press.

Kripke, S. (1963). Semantical considerations on modal logic. *Acta Philosophica Fennica, 16,* 83–94.

Leibniz, G. W. (1710/1985). *Theodicy: Essays on the goodness of God, the freedom on man and the origin of evil* (E. M. Huggard, Trans.). La Salle, IL: Open Court.

Leslie, A. M. (1987). Pretense and representation: The origins of "theory of mind". *Psychological Review, 94,* 412–426.

Lyon, D. R., Gunzelmann, G., & Gluck, K. A. (2008). A computational model of spatial visualization capacity. *Cognitive Psychology, 57,* 122–152.

McDonough, I. M., & Gallo, D. A. (2010). Separating past and future autobiographical events in memory: Evidence for a reality monitoring asymmetry. *Memory & Cognition, 38*(1), 3–12.

Mitroff, S. R., Scholl, B. J., & Wynn, K. (2005). The relationship between object files and conscious perception. *Cognition, 96,* 67–92.

Nardini, M., Thomas, R. L., Knowland, V. C. P., Braddick, O. J., & Atkinson, J. (2009). A viewpoint-independent process for spatial reorientation. *Cognition, 112,* 241–248.

Nash, R. A., Wade, K. A., & Lindsay, D. S. (2009). Digitally manipulating memory: Effects of doctored videos and imagination in distorting beliefs and memories. *Memory & Cognition, 37*(4), 414–424.

Newman, E. G., Choi, H., Wynn, K., & Scholl, B. J. (2008). The origins of causal perception: Evidence from postdictive processing in infancy. *Cognitive Psychology, 57,* 262–291.

Plagnol, A. (1993). *Elaboration d'un modèle de désorganisation des représentations mentales par décontextualisation fonctionnelle de l'information* [A model of disorganization of mental representations by functional decontextualization] (Unpublished doctoral dissertation). Orsay, France: Université Paris 11.

Plagnol, A. (2002). La structure pliée des espaces de représentation: théorie élémentaire. *Intellectica, 35,* 27–81.

Plagnol, A. (2004). *Espaces de représentation: Théorie élémentaire et psychopathologie* [Representational spaces: Elements and psychopathology]. Paris: Editions du CNRS.

Plagnol, A. (in press). *Principes de navigation dans les mondes possibles* [Principles of navigation in possible worlds]. Garches, France: Terra Cotta.

Plagnol, A., Pachoud, B., Claudel, B., & Granger, B. (1996). Functional disorganization of representations in schizophrenia. *Schizophrenia Bulletin, 22*(2), 383–404.

Platek, S. M., & Shackelford, T. M. (2009). *Foundations in evolutionary cognitive neuroscience.* Cambridge: Cambridge University Press.

Potts, G. R., & Peterson, S. B. (1985). Incorporation versus compartmentalization in memory for discourse. *Journal of Memory and Language, 24,* 107–118.

Potts, G. R., St. John, M. F., & Kirson, D. (1989). Incorporating new information into existing world knowledge. *Cognitive Psychology, 21,* 303–333.

Preminger, O. (1954). *River of no return* [Film]. Los Angeles, CA: 20th Century Fox.

Ragni, M., & Knauff, M. (2013). A theory and a computational model of spatial reasoning with preferred mental models. *Psychological Review, 120*(3), 561–588.

Rubin, D. C., & Umanath, S. (2015). Event memory: A theory of memory for laboratory, autobiographical and fictional events. *Psychological Review, 122*(1), 1–23.

Scott, R. M., Baillargeon, R., Song, H., & Leslie, A. M. (2010). Attributing false beliefs about non-obvious properties at 18 months. *Cognitive Psychology, 61,* 366–395.

Soto, D., Wriglesworth, A., Bahrami-Balani, A., & Humphreys, G. W. (2010). Working memory enhances visual perception: Evidence from signal detection analysis. *Journal of Experimental Psychology: Learning, Memory, and Cognition, 36*(2), 441–456.

Zaragoza, M. S., Mitchell, K. J., Payment, K., & Drivdahl, S. (2011). False memories for suggestions: The impact of conceptual elaboration. *Journal of Memory and Language, 64,* 18–31.

10

Two Paradigms to Explore Inner Worlds: Spatial and Fictional Navigation

1   Introduction

In the previous chapter, we laid the cognitive foundations for an approach of inner worlds and navigation in possible worlds. These advances in cognitive science allow us to develop the scientific study of domains fundamental to mental activity, as we will show by first studying two target fields: mental travel in material space and fictional worlds.

In this chapter, we specify the basic tools that make it possible to account for our ability to navigate mentally in space or fiction, and we highlight their interest both in deepening the understanding of mental distress and in enriching the therapeutic arsenal (or to better justify care methods already widely used). In Chapter 11, the paradigmatic value of these two target domains will become apparent, as we will use the same fundamental concepts introduced in this chapter to address the "high level" navigation involved in understanding others and in the scientific, aesthetic and spiritual domains.

© The Author(s) 2019
T. Ward and A. Plagnol, *Cognitive Psychodynamics as an Integrative Framework in Counselling Psychology and Psychotherapy*,
https://doi.org/10.1007/978-3-030-25823-8_10

2   Spatial Travel

Mind travel in space ("spatial travel") is a first fundamental domain where our navigation capabilities are at work in an internal universe. We recognize this implicitly when we consider such a universe as a representational *space* or when we use the metaphor of mental *navigation*. This metaphor does not date from the Internet but was already dear to Plato![1] In fact, we use an infinite number of spatial metaphors in everyday language to evoke our psychological sensations.

Let's take a few examples in pathology: a depressed client talks about "low mood", "fall" or "dark well"; a person experiencing mania seems to "take off" or "glide"; someone with schizophrenia suggests that their universe is "fragmented"; or, in psychotherapy, we say of a client that he "travels a path", that he "opens a door", that he "makes a step". According to the founder of existential analysis [*Daseinanalyse*], Ludwig Binswanger, essential structures underlie such metaphors (Binswanger, 1930/1963).

> Binswanger (1930/1963, 1947) stressed the anthropological dimension of *verticality*: the possibility of *ascension*, even of *flight* and *fall*, would be an essential feature of human presence in the world. According to Binswanger, the *presumption/extravagance* [*Verstiegenheit*] is revealed by some "discordance" between the vertical momentum and the horizontal displacement (Binswanger, 1949/1963, 1958/1989). The presumption can "lead astray in the heights" or towards a *deadlock*, when an overly ideal momentum has taken the subject away. For example, Binswanger analysed the inner world of a person experiencing mania from this perspective: *speed, leap, take-off, levelling of space* are cardinal determinations of such a world (Binswanger, 1933; Plagnol, 2003, 2004). *Verstiegen* refers precisely to the situation of a blocked mountaineer who can no longer make a movement without the help of others. Psychotherapy, like a rescue line to the mountaineer in distress, has as its founding aim to bring the subject *back to earth* (Binswanger, 1958/1989).

Binswanger's phenomenological insights are now supported by the development of the conceptual framework of the *embodied cognition*,

---

[1]See, for example, Plato's *Phaedo* 99d, *Statesman* 300c, *Philebus* 19c.

which is based on extensive experimental research showing how any representation is rooted in spatialized sensorimotor patterns (Glenberg, 1997).[2] Lakoff and Johnson (1999), with their famous theory of *conceptual metaphors*, also confirmed that the use of language, even in its most abstract aspects, is based on spatio-temporal categories.

Such a perspective is not only relevant for advanced laboratory research. Being able to imagine an alternative path—for example, for foraging or war—confers a considerable evolutionary advantage, and this decisive leap in possible worlds must have been present for the human species since prehistoric times.

The skills to navigate virtually in space are practiced on a daily basis, for example, when we have to plan a trip to the station. The alteration of these skills is an important aspect of the functional impact of certain pathologies marked by withdrawal, such as depression, agoraphobia or schizophrenia. The daily outcome of ageing is also characterized by a progressive restriction on the possibilities of spatial travel—a restriction that is tragically increased in Alzheimer's disease, for which impairments in spatial navigation are one of the earliest cognitive deficits (Allison, Fagan, Morris, & Head, 2016).

After having specified some elementary processes that underlie mental navigation in space, we will consider the potential contribution of such navigation to the treatment of a series of psychologically distressing conditions.

2.1 Elementary Cognitive Processes

As we have seen in the preceding chapter, to move in space mentally, for example, to plan a journey, we must *construct paths*, i.e. link limited views (snapshots/scenes) in our presence window through *symbolic structures*.[3]

---

[2]The embodied cognition framework can be integrated into the broader framework of *grounded cognition* (Barsalou, 2008), for which symbolic representations rely on iconic/analogical representations to receive content (see Chapter 9, Sect. 2.1).

[3]See the example of virtual walks in London, Chapter 9, Sect. 2.1, and the definition of symbolic structures in Chapter 9, Sect. 2.3.

We are familiar with such exercises and we can even say that we are virtuosos of space navigation: we can move mentally at high speed in spaces as varied as our home, our city, the Earth… by changing scale at an amazing speed. The elementary skills that underlie such virtuosity are exercised when using Google Maps® software or GPS navigation instruments, which necessarily work with the same basic principles as the human mind.

2.1.1 Globalization and Focusing

We prioritize the elements of space according to flexible "categories" (Ferguson & Hegarty, 1994; Greenauer & Waller, 2010; Holden, Curby, Newcombe, & Shipley, 2010; Hutcheson & Wedell, 2009, Uttal, Friedman, Hand, & Warren, 2010). Based on this hierarchical structure, two symmetrical processes are at work in rapid changes of scale:

- *Globalization* is the deployment of an abstract view condensing a set of scenes/snapshots. Indeed, we can develop "mental maps" or abstract representations that directly deploy global spatial relationships (Levine, Jankovic, & Palij, 1982; Plagnol, in press; Thorndyke & Hayes-Roth, 1982; Trope & Liberman, 2010). Such representations make it possible to see "at a glance" (in the presence window) the route to be taken.
- *Focusing* is the projection of a scene/snapshot from a global view. A focus is often based on a *landmark*, public (river, monument…) or personal (linked to a subjective story, such as the school of his/her childhood). Landmarks can be used as *anchor points* for connecting a mental map to real material space and as *seed data* for locating other points (Friedman & Brown, 2000; Plagnol, 2007, in press). The activation of the landmark's name functions as a tab on a mental map (Nardini, Thomas, Knowland, Braddick, & Atkinson, 2009; Newman et al., 2007; Ruddle, Volkova, Mohler, & Bülthoff, 2011). For example, if a friend tells us on the phone that they are in Hyde Park, near the Albert Memorial, we can mentally deploy a global map of Hyde Park and then focus on the Albert Memorial from our mental node *Albert Memorial*.

2.1.2 Flexibility

We seldom realize how easy it is to move around in a familiar space like our home or neighbourhood. Indeed, in such cases, reinforced symbolic structures allow us to quickly link the fragments we need in our presence window. If Tom the Londoner has to cross Hyde Park every day from Kensington Palace to Marble Arch on his way to work, he can easily reconstruct mentally his journey.

However, we often have to put new symbolic structures into action to achieve new goals. Let's take our last example again and suppose that Tom has to anticipate a detour to Hyde Park Corner on a beautiful Sunday morning for a first romantic date. In this case, Tom can easily find a new mental path from Kensington Palace to Marble Arch through Hyde Park Corner: he just needs to deploy a mental plan of Hyde Park (using the help of an external map if necessary), to visualize a path globally and to activate symbolic items like *Albert Memorial* or *Knightsbridge* to focus on the important steps. Subsequently, each opening of this path will strengthen the symbolic structure that connects the different snapshots that make it up, so that Tom can travel this path faster and faster—for example, if Tom likes to delightfully retrace the details of his first romantic date—just as a path in the forest widens as the walkers pass by.[4]

In this example, the activation of a goal ("Hyde Park Corner") changes the functional memory context and influences Tom's choice of path to Marble Arch. In general, the dynamic properties of the activation network that constitute the mental web allow a great flexibility, the weight of the links between symbolic items being permanently modulated by the functional memory context, i.e. the distribution of the activation in the network.

In particular, the "vertical" links hierarchizing spatial areas and allowing globalization/focusing operations depend on the functional

---

[4]Conversely, a mental path that is not taken can become so difficult to practice that it leads nowhere because its symbolic structure is gradually erased, like a *Holzweg* in the Black Forest (Heidegger 1950/1994; Plagnol, 2004)—such phenomena may be common in Alzheimer's disease (Delrue & Plagnol, 2017; Plagnol, in press).

memory context, resulting in high flexibility in spatial categorizations (Hutcheson & Wedell, 2009; Uttal et al., 2010). For example, the memory node *Kensington Palace* can activate the node *Hyde Park* in the context of a walk in the famous park, or the node *Kensington* in the context of a walk in Kensington, or directly the "higher" node *London* in the context of a visit to the capital...[5]

We can also very easily *change our perspective* by taking into account contextual information. For example, we have surprising flexibility to consider alternative views of the same location (Brunyé, Rapp, & Taylor, 2008; Meilinger, Berthoz, & Wiener, 2011; Waller, Friedman, Hodgson, & Greenauer, 2009). If you are a Londoner, you can probably easily position yourself mentally at Oxford Circus from several points of view—imagine that you arrive at Oxford Circus by Oxford Street first from the west then from the east, then by Regent Street first from the north then from the south. From the age of five, a child is able to remember a place although not put in a perspective that he/she has not yet experienced (Nardini et al., 2009).

2.2   Form Material Space to the Mental Universe

Whatever the field, only one method is possible to navigate in a mental universe: to deploy in a limited presence window a series of snapshots/scenes/mental models linked by symbolic structures, i.e. *to forge paths*. The art of mental navigation is thus based on the ability to structure a field in a relevant way, with the same basic tools as for navigation in material space:

- Abstract models allow *globalization*, i.e. the deployment of globalized contents in the presence window;

---

[5]The compartmentalization we introduced in the previous chapter, concerning the representation of possible worlds, is a case of rigid contextualization. Let us note that our partitions of space are sometimes compartments: if you have always stayed in Europe, it is possible that your mental China functions as a world different from your usual world. (The very rare Latin authors who mention the existence of China ("*Seres*") conceived it as a world different from their world.)

- Symbolic units, when activated, allow *focusing*, i.e. the deployment of targeted contents in the presence window. Such *retrieval cues* have long been proposed in experimental psychology (Anderson, 1983; Clifton & Slowiaczek, 1981; Potts & Peterson, 1985; Reder & Ross, 1983).

Schemas (Rumelhart, 1975), *retrieval structures* (Ericsson & Kintsch, 1995), or *script*s (Raisig, Welke, Hagendorf, & van der Meer, 2009) show the cognitive value of reinforced symbolic fragments allowing rapid navigation in a specific field of competence.

However, flexibility is essential to allow new paths to be opened when faced with new tasks (e.g. van Elk, van Schie, & Bekkering, 2009). The flexibility of memory—memories are reconstructed according to a "projective" and contextualized process—favours its essential orientation towards the future (Berntsen & Bohn, 2010; Hassabis & Maguire, 2007; Schacter, Addis, & Buckner, 2008; Suddendorf & Corballis, 2007; Szpunar, 2010).

Not only does mental spatial navigation involve capacities that are constantly used in daily life, but the dynamics of the inner world as a whole are largely based on the same type of capacities: orientation, changes of scale/context, globalization and focusing, functional contextualization, changes of perspective, flexibility of symbolic structures. Spatial mental navigation therefore offers a stimulating paradigm for clinical work, as we will now show by detailing a few examples.

2.3   Phobia

In Chapter 8, we highlighted the usefulness of therapeutic levers, i.e. situations that can mobilize the entire inner universe from the work done in the therapeutic space.

Virtual navigation in space offers rich possibilities for forging such levers:

- This is naturally the case in phobias where material space is directly involved, as in agoraphobia, and most effective therapeutic techniques now use virtual reality navigation (Botella, Fernández-Alvarez, Gillén, Garcia-Palacios, & Baños, 2017). Desensitization by immersion in imaginary situations is in fact already a form of navigation in possible worlds!

- By rigorously basing it on the cognitive foundations of space navigation, it becomes possible to propose work as close as possible to the agoraphobic syndrome with regard to its hold on the inner world. For example, virtual routes to a chosen destination can be systematically varied, the client can be taught how to use his/her mental maps flexibly by alternating globalization and focusing or to plan reassuring landmarks and anchor points.

- The work on space navigation is not only interesting for agoraphobia. Indeed, any phobia is defined by a specific external situation, and the loss of autonomy is defined in terms of the restriction of accessible space. Above all, a phobic situation reflects the structure of the inner world by materializing the dimensions that make it vulnerable (Chapter 8, Sect. 2.3). For example, in elevator phobia, the characteristic dimensions are *foundations instability, lack of way out, speed* and *penetrance*: all these dimensions can be addressed from material space situations, especially using virtual reality devices.

- Table 1 in Chapter 8 makes it easy to conceive, for each type of phobia, how work on mental trajectories can provide a lever targeting the dimensions of vulnerability of the inner world underlying the phobic situation, without excessive emotional risk.

- Such work can be further developed by fostering a progressive metacognition of the relationship between the dimensions of vulnerability and the phobic situation, in order to address phobogenic schemas and facilitate a comprehensive restructuring of the inner world.[6]

---

[6]More targeted work can use the home metaphor and its different dimensions to address the Home ideal and make the link with situations from childhood. The ocean metaphor (Chapter 8, Sect. 3) can also give rise to spatial navigation work.

2.4   Depression

We have already emphasized the multiple spatial metaphors that are common to describe the phenomenology of depression: "confinement", "lack of escape", "withdrawal", "fall"... The "well" metaphor, often expressed by clients, highlights the experience associated with the risk of relapse, any attempt to escape from the depressive state inducing a wave of pain.[7] The psychomotor slowing observed in severe depressive episodes directly reflects the *retraction* of the inner world (Plagnol, 2004).

A work on space navigation can again be relevant to remobilize psychic life without putting the subject in danger of relapse: material space is a relatively emotionally neutral medium and can even offer encounters that reopen the mental space in an unexpected way. Binswanger (1960) reported the case of a melancholic subject leaving Privatsanatorium Bellevue to hang himself in the Black Forest, but who regained a taste for life when a cute little weasel ran off into the glade!

By softly mobilizing mental space navigation, it is possible to:

- work on virtual outings even though the subject is confined to his/ her house or even his/her room;
- consider alternative routes, changes of perspective, discovery of potential landmarks and anchor points;
- work on the concept of globalization and focusing, as a first step to soften cognitive distortions often at the heart of depressogenic thinking schemas (Beck, Rush, Shaw, & Emery, 1989);
- constitute the therapeutic framework as a "safe place", with the space it opens up and that the subject can freely appropriate within his/her inner world;
- gradually, and after ensuring that the therapeutic framework is sufficiently solid, metaphorically address the tears, cracks and flaws of the inner world.

---

[7]See Chapter 6, Sect. 5.

2.5   Obsessive-Compulsive Conditions

Severe obsessive-compulsive syndromes are often marked by a considerable restriction of the material space accessible to the subject, due to obsessive thoughts and rituals. For example, the subject may be entirely confined to the house or even to a part of his/her room to avoid any risk of contamination, a major part of his/her ordinary space being "taboo".[8] And even in obsessive-compulsive disorders where the material space is not directly restricted by pathology, the accessible world is impoverished because any material or mental path must be rigidly demarcated, within a wholly standardized control space.

As we saw in Chapter 8, in an obsessive syndrome, the power of fantasy—that is, the ability to navigate through the possible worlds—is paradoxically turned against the subject himself by a near equal power of symbolic control. For example, the fantasy of contamination by a microbe develops into a catastrophic thought (contamination of the Home in particular) and the subject must "erase" the obsessive intrusion by a ritual of equal power. Therefore, how can we rely on the capacities of the subject himself, so that he succeeds in putting at his/her service both his fantasy power and his/her control power rather than shearing himself by this double scythe?

Here again, working on a virtual material space offers a relatively neutral field where the client can become aware that navigating through the possible worlds is without real danger. It may therefore be useful to propose to the client to:

- build virtual reality models corresponding to obsessions-compulsions (not necessarily those of the client to begin with);
- in this virtual space, develop a "fearsome" situation through increasingly precise projections/focalizations so that the client can tolerate "disasters"—for example, contact and stain—that are more and more intense and widespread (and even accept the paradoxical pleasure provided by them);

---

[8]See the case of Miss J in Chapter 8, Sect. 4.

- propose exercises in functional compartmentalization/decompartmentalization to put into perspective the true meaning of borders and taboo areas;
- teach the subject to play with symbolic structures, landmarks and ritualized mental paths to gradually release their hold;
- in general, help the subject to allow himself to play, fantasize, navigate in the possible worlds and discover by metacognition all his/her resources at his/her disposal for this navigation; and
- once a solid therapeutic framework has been established and control has begun to relax, explore the metaphorical value of the condition in relation to the inner world (e.g. the problem of a stain in a home can lead to an understanding of the problem of the stain in the Home).

2.6   Schizophrenia

Impairments in spatial navigation have been evidenced in schizophrenia and could be related to key functional neurobiological characteristics associated with this condition (Daniel, Dibio-Cohen, Carité, Boyer, & Denis, 2007; Siddiqui et al., 2018; Zawadzki et al., 2013). Many clients have difficulties in daily travel, and transportation use is one main component of functional capacity assessment in these disorders (Mausbach, Harvey, Goldman, Jeste, & Patterson, 2007; Ruse et al., 2014). Functional capacity training programmes include significant elements for spatial navigation, frequently through simulation or virtual reality modules (e.g. Amado et al., 2016).

Beyond reducing neurocognitive difficulties and improving daily autonomy, mental navigation in material space can be used to address the pathogenic processes themselves as they are reflected in the (de) structuring of the inner world. Indeed, schizophrenia is classically described as personality *fragmentation* (or *splitting*) [*Spaltung*], with a *withdrawal* on the inner world (Bleuler, 1911/1950; Plagnol, 2004). Fragmentation and withdrawal are spatial metaphors that reflect what is at the heart of schizophrenia, namely a vicious circle between the fragmentation forces in the inner world and the defensive tendency to withdraw. Areas excluded from subject consciousness by denial processes function as interfering parasitic zones (Plagnol, 2004; Plagnol, Oïta, Montreuil, Granger, & Lubart, 2003—see also Fig. 4 in Chapter 9). This leads to a general blurring of the structure of the mental space responsible for most symptoms of incoherence.

Virtual navigation in space thus offers rich possibilities for the client to work on his/her inner world:

- The construction of virtual spaces allows, for example, of flexible compartmentalization and to explain the interest of landmarks or anchor points.
- The initiation of metacognition through greater control of space can help to regain control, which is the first step in a recovery process.
- The fragmentation process, the impact of parasitic areas, etc., can be understood in a spatialized form.

Mrs. P, 54, has been followed by the community centre for more than 20 years because of schizophrenia. She does not leave her home, except for her monthly meeting at the clinic. The nurse who regularly makes home visits is alarmed by the accumulation of objects and waste, indicative of a hoarding disorder. Neighbours complain about smells and health risks. During an interview, her therapist tries to discuss the hoarding's problem with Mrs. P, talking about a link with her illness. To the surprise of the therapist, Mrs. P asks what her illness is. The therapist understands that Mrs. P is asking less for a diagnosis than for appropriate explanations about her condition.

The therapist sketches a rough diagram of the "brain", draws "parasitic zones", explains that these zones are generally linked to difficult events of the past that are removed from the memory because they are too painful, tries to show with arrows the fragmentations that such parasitic zones cause, the interferences in memory and the overload of the mental space. In fact, it reproduces a schema similar to Fig. 4 in Chapter 9, a schema that has little to do with true neurological structures but expresses the structure of Mrs. P's inner world as he sees it. The therapist then has the insight of a parallel between the accumulation of objects in Mrs. P's home and the overload of her inner world, which he allows himself to formulate with a smile to Mrs. P. She too smiles, shows great interest, and thanks for the explanations given.

> At the next home visit, the nurse is very surprised: Mrs. P tidied up her apartment a little. Mrs. P is even able to allow the nurse to take away bags that had been smelling strongly for a long time. In the next weeks and months, Mrs. P began to leave her home, visit museums, reconnect with family members and even take trips. Not only is her home cleaned, but her inner world seems to have been renovated, along with the spectacular extension of her range in space, as well as of her exchanges with the outside world.

3   Fictional Travel

A second paradigmatic domain for navigation in possible worlds is constituted by situations where an alternative world to the real world is built according to specific rules: games, novels, theatre plays and films.

We have an astonishing ability to immerse ourselves in artificial worlds, sometimes inspired by the real world, sometimes completely freeing ourselves from it. The ability to immerse oneself in a fictional world is so essential to human beings that all oral traditions are mainly the transmission of myths, that the first significant written trace—*The Epic of Gilgamesh* (Anonymous Babylonian poets, from 3700 BC to twenty-first century BC/2003)—is fictional, and that a small child, barely sketching out his/her first words, plunges into the delights of pretence (from 18 months).

Whilst these fictional worlds are sometimes very simple, such as a scene told one evening to a 2-year-old child, they can also be very complex, as suggested by the example of children's stories in Chapter 9: nested within each other, intertwined with "epistemic" worlds attributed to characters (see the example of Snow White and the Witch in Chapter 9, Sect. 3.1) or woven with "temporal" worlds that immerse us in other eras for our delight such as when we read *Quentin Durward* (Scott, 1823/2011) or *The Three Musketeers* (Dumas, 1844/2008).

Such constructions reveal the limitless pleasure that a human being can take in imitating the real world and liberating him/herself from it, in inventing rules to build a universe, in immersing him/herself in unknown worlds built by others, in exploring such worlds and returning from them, in extending and refining them and, last but not least, in sharing such discoveries.

Fictional navigation is now enriched by the formidable means offered by virtual reality techniques, electronic consoles and the Internet, which allow highly sophisticated narrative games or online games combining almost unlimited numbers of players (MMORPGs).[9]

3.1   Elementary Cognitive Processes

Spatial travel, studied in Sect. 2, can be considered as a special case of fictional travel—many games are based on virtual exploration of the material world or on mental simulation of trajectories (e.g. chess). Of course, unlike the "simple" spatial travel, fictional travel, by inventing objects and introducing specific laws, makes it possible to free oneself from the constraints of the real world. However, the same principles as those we have considered for mental navigation in physical space apply. Indeed, it is always a task of presenting scenes/snapshots in a narrow window of presence and linking them with symbolic structures. Let us specify some key processes that underlie navigation in fictional universes:

- The fictional worlds are compartmentalized from the real world, as are the different fictional worlds between them, i.e. the contents deployed are tagged as belonging to one world or another (see Chapter 9, Sect. 3.3). This compartmentalization is in principle functional and flexible enough to allow mental comings and goings between immersion in fiction and return to reality. In practice, navigation in fictional worlds may require use of sophisticated pointers to ensure the nesting of worlds, the entanglements with epistemic or temporal aspects, and the dynamic differentiation of replicas (counterparts/avatars) from one world to another. Consider, for example, the representational complexity involved in reading a novel such as *The Ambassadors* (James, 1903/2008): each character has an inner

---

[9]Massively multiplayer online role-playing games.

world of great richness, representing the worlds of the other characters and developing his/her own subjective replica of Paris at the beginning of the twentieth century.

- Symbolic structures are forged to "store" in memory the fragments not available in the presence window or to chain fragments in the presence window when they are reactivated. For example, when reading a fictional narrative that is not limited to a single scene, we cannot deploy the entire universe represented in our presence window, hence, the use of *retrieval structures*: elements that are not deployed at a given time are stored in long-term memory and reactivated according to their links to active items in working memory (Ericsson & Kintsch, 1995; Gernsbacher, Varner, & Faust, 1990; Graesser, Singer, & Trabasso, 1994; Zwaan & Radvansky, 1998).

- To enable rapid navigation, symbolic structures associated with a fictional world are often rigidified in the form of schemas (Rumelhart, 1975) or scripts (Raisig et al., 2009). Similarly, an expert player in a field is able to use tactical patterns very quickly, which allows him/her to effectively chart mental paths to win. However, creativity also requires flexibility to allow changes of perspective—for example, some chess studies have shown that grand masters are able to free themselves from tactical patterns if necessary, contrary to "simple" experts (Bilalić, McLeod, & Gobet, 2008).

- The symbolic structures associated with fiction also allow for globalization and focusing operations. Indeed, we need both models to "synthesize" the action and projections to target some details. Graesser et al. (1994) showed that a reader organizes local information chunks into global chunks, whilst the explanation of some details (i.e. focusing) depends on his/her objectives. A novel thus alternates global considerations on the plot framework with detailed scenes; similarly, a chess player alternates global strategic insights with tactical projections.

- Finally, the organization of symbolic structures into hierarchical networks provides contextual nodes and landmarks that facilitate tracking in a fictional world. Indeed, such a task can be tricky when it concerns a world that is at first unknown, sometimes extended in multiple episodes, with returns to the past or projections into the future, such as the sagas of *Star Wars* (Lucas, 1977–2005) or *Harry*

Potter (Rowling, 1997–2007). A fiction writer or director, if they are concerned not to misplace their readers/viewers too much, sows enough clues so that they always know where they are.

3.2   Fiction and Therapy

The interest of fictional travel in psychotherapy is commensurate with our prodigious capacities for mental navigation in fictional worlds. These universes can be adjusted as closely as possible to the client's inner world and what he or she can bear, in a dynamic relationship with another person within a therapeutic framework. Let us highlight some aspects of fictional travel that may be particularly useful from a clinical perspective:

- Mediation of the emotions through an adapted framework, circumscribed by compartmentalization as an imaginary space;
- Exploration of emotionally charged situations with an infinite number of possible nuances. Indeed, the whole range of human emotions can be reflected in fiction;
- Discovery of the mental worlds of characters with their own beliefs and emotions. Differences in subjective perspectives, and more broadly in inner worlds, can thus be safely grasped;
- Exploration of new worlds, allowing to reopen new horizons. Using projective imagination skills can be particularly interesting when they are curbed, for example, in depression, obsessive conditions or schizophrenia;
- Discovery of the pleasure of building a coherent world, of gradually structuring it, of tracing paths and crossing it based on landmarks, of finally mastering it to the point of being able to navigate it at high speed and of inviting other subjects to share it;
- Uncovering of creative resources that enrich the subject's metacognition and improves their self-esteem;
- Proposal of models for the construction of a life history, that is the "backbone" of the inner world. In particular, fictional narratives or narrative games, with the misfortunes and resilience paths of the characters, provide rich identification tools to integrate the hardships and traumas of life into a more unified personal story.

The construction of a life story by the client, or rather its co-construction with the therapist, is often considered a pillar of psychotherapy. Many therapeutic paradigms nowadays have a strong narrative dimension based on the tools of cognitive science. For example, there is a blossoming of *life review therapies* and *reminiscence therapies* under multiple conditions: dementia (Park, Lee, Yang, & Song, 2019), cancer patients (Zhang, Xiao, & Chen, 2017), schizophrenia (Chen et al., 2017).

Such narrative therapies involve the *mental time travel* ability (Michaelian, 2016; Suddendorf & Corballis, 2007; Tulving, 2002), that is, the ability to project into the past or the future. Mental time travel, based on episodic memory, can be regarded as combining space travel and fictional travel: on the one hand, a time *travel* can only be represented in a spatialized way, as the paradigm of embodied cognition insists (see Casasanto & Boroditsky, 2008); on the other hand, a time travel is always fictional, given that memory is always a reconstruction oriented to the future (see Sect. 2.2) and that anticipation of the future ("episodic future thinking") is by nature fictional. Since Tulving's pioneering work on episodic memory (Tulving, 1985, 2002), mental time travel has become a hot topic in cognitive science research, inspiring many clinical applications (see Michaelian, 2016; Michaelian, Klein, & Szpunar, 2016).

The immense possibilities offered by fictional travel have of course been used for a long time, both in clinical evaluation and psychotherapy. Fundamental in the approach to children—let us limit ourselves to recalling the major work of Donald Winnicott (e.g. Winnicott, 1971/2005)—fictional travel also serves as a basis for many therapeutic techniques in adults—play, theatre, writing, etc., which can be combined in countless variants. The resources of fictional travel are exploited far beyond the realm of mental health, as evidenced by the development of the narrative-medicine (Charon et al., 2016; Greenhalgh & Hurwitz, 1999; Roberts, 2000), and even play a significant role in the training of health care personal (fictional case studies, role plays, awareness of the narrative aspects of care...).

All therapeutic techniques based on fictional travel are today profoundly renewed by the fascinating development of electronic simulation tools, including virtual reality devices, which constantly open new horizons for clinicians. To take just one example, "serious games" for autistic people (long considered to be unable to play) have become a very dynamic area of clinical practice—a recent meta-analysis by Grossard et al. (2017) identifies no less than 31 serious games targeting social skills in autism spectrum disorders!

Such a proliferation makes it all the more pressing to build a framework in which the different therapeutic techniques using fictional travel can be described in an integrated way, their specificities mapped out, their effectiveness assessed in a comparative manner and their indications clarified. We take the reasonable bet that such a framework will be, in one way or another, cognitive psychodynamic.

4   Concluding Remarks

Cognitive science research on space travel and fictional travel can provide a more solid scientific basis for many therapies that have used such tools for a long time but have often remained quite intuitive. Advances in cognitive science also make it possible to envisage much more targeted work according to the subjects' inner worlds, especially since new technical tools, such as those offered by virtual reality, now multiply the possibilities of creating tailor-made clinical settings.

Some therapeutic techniques based on fictional travel are already undergoing spectacular developments. We may think that we are still in the early stages of the scientific design of these tools, which will be enriched in the very near future. It is all the more important to develop a cognitive-psychodynamic approach that is sufficiently refined to provide a framework that could integrate all the contributions of these tools and feed their development in a clinically relevant way.

We will see in the next chapter that the therapeutic contributions of fictional travel and spatial travel can extend to the most prestigious fields of human activity.

References

Allison, S. L., Fagan, A. M., Morris, J. C., & Head, D. (2016). Spatial navigation in preclinical Alzheimer's disease. *Journal of Alzheimer's Disease, 52*(1), 77–90.

Amado, I., Brénugat-Herné, L., Orriols, E., Desombre, C., Dos Santos, M., Prost, Z., ... Piolino, P. (2016, April 20). A serious game to improve cognitive functions in schizophrenia: A pilot study. *Frontiers in Psychiatry*. Retrieved February 24, 2019, from https://doi.org/10.3389/fpsyt.2016.00064.

Anderson, J. R. (1983). *The architecture of cognition*. Cambridge, MA: Harvard University Press.

Anonymous Babylonian poets. (From 3700 BC to 21st century BC/2003). *The epic of gilgamesh* (A. George, Trans.). London: Penguin Classics.

Barsalou, L. W. (2008). Grounded cognition. *Annual Review of Psychology, 59*, 617–645.

Beck, A., Rush, A. J., Shaw, B. F., & Emery, G. (1989). *Cognitive therapy of depression*. New York: Guilford.

Berntsen, D., & Bohn, A. (2010). Remembering and forecasting: The relation between autobiographical memory and episodic future thinking. *Memory & Cognition, 38*(3), 265–278.

Bilalić, M., McLeod, P., & Gobet, F. (2008). Why good thoughts block better ones: The mechanism of the pernicious Einstellung (set) effect. *Cognition, 108*, 652–661.

Binswanger, L. (1930/1963). Dream and existence. In L. Binswanger (Ed.), *Being-in-the-world: Selected papers of Ludwig Binswanger* (J. Needleman, Trans., pp. 222–248). New York: Basic Books.

Binswanger, L. (1933). *Über Ideenflucht* [On 'idea escape']. Zurich: Orell-Füssli.

Binswanger, L. (1947). Bemerkungen zu zwei wenig beachteten "Gedanken" pascals über Symmetrie [Remarks on two little-noticed "thoughts" of Pascal about symmetry]. *Zeitschrift Für Kinderpsychiatrie, 14*, 19–27.

Binswanger, L. (1949/1963). Extravagance (Verstiegenheit). In L. Binswanger (Ed.), *Being-in-the-world: Selected papers of Ludwig Binswanger* (J. Needleman, Trans., pp. 342–349). New York: Basic Books.

Binswanger, L. (1958/1989). Analyse existentielle et psychothérapie (II). In L. Binswanger (Ed.), *Introduction à l'analyse existentielle* [Introduction to existential analysis] (J. Verdaux & R. Kuhn, Trans., pp. 149–157). Paris: Minuit.

Binswanger, L. (1960). *Melancholie und Manie: Phänomenologische Studien* [Melancholy and mania: Phenomenological studies]. Pfullingen, Germany: Günther Neske.

Bleuler, E. (1911/1950). *Dementia praecox or the group of schizophrenias* (J. Zinkin, Trans.). New York: International Universities Press.

Botella, C., Fernández-Alvarez, J., Gillén, V., Garcia-Palacios, A., & Baños, R. (2017). Recent progress in virtual reality exposure therapy for phobias: A systematic review. *Current Psychiatry Reports, 19*(7), 42. https://doi.org/10.1007/s11920-017-0788-4.

Brunyé, T. T., Rapp, D. N., & Taylor, H. A. (2008). Representational flexibility and specificity following spatial descriptions of real-world environments. *Cognition, 108,* 418–443.

Casasanto, D., & Boroditsky, L. (2008). Time in the mind: Using space to think about time. *Cognition, 106*(2), 579–593.

Charon, R., DasGupta, S., Hermann, N., Irvine, C., Marcus, E. R., Colón, E. R., ... Spiegel, M. (2016). *The Principles and practice of narrative medicine.* New York: Oxford University Press.

Chen, G.-F., Liu, L.L., Cui, J.-F., Chen, T., Qin, X.-J., Gan, J.-C., ... Chan, R. C. K. (2017). Life review therapy enhances mental time travel in patients with schizophrenia. *Psychiatry Research, 258,* 145–152.

Clifton, C., Jr., & Slowiaczek, M. L. (1981). Integrating new information with old knowledge. *Memory & Cognition, 9,* 142–148.

Daniel, M.-P., Dibio-Cohen, C. M., Carité, L., Boyer, P., & Denis, M. (2007). Dysfunctions of spatial cognition in schizophrenic patients. *Spatial Cognition and Computation, 7*(3), 287–309.

Delrue, N., & Plagnol, A. (2017). Post-traumatic stress disorder in Alzheimer's disease. *Counselling Psychology Review, 32*(4), 58–69.

Dumas, A. (1844/2008). *The three musketeers* (R. Pevear, Trans.). London: Penguin Classics.

Ericsson, K. A., & Kintsch, W. (1995). Long-term working memory. *Psychological Review, 102,* 211–245.

Ferguson, E. L., & Hegarty, M. (1994). Properties of cognitive maps constructed from texts. *Memory & Cognition, 22,* 455–473.

Friedman, A., & Brown, N. R. (2000). Updating geographical knowledge: Principles of coherence and inertia. *Journal of Experimental Psychology: Learning, Memory, and Cognition, 26*(4), 900–914.

Gernsbacher, M. A., Varner, K. R., & Faust, M. E. (1990). Investigating differences in general comprehension skill. *Journal of Experimental Psychology: Learning, Memory, and Cognition, 16,* 430–445.

Glenberg, A. M. (1997). What memory is for. *Behavioral and Brain Sciences, 20,* 1–55.

Graesser, A. C., Singer, M., & Trabasso, T. (1994). Constructing inferences during narrative text comprehension. *Psychological Review, 101,* 371–395.

Greenauer, N., & Waller, D. (2010). Micro- and macroreference frames: Specifying the relations between spatial categories in memory. *Journal of Experimental Psychology: Learning, Memory, and Cognition, 36*(4), 938–957.

Greenhalgh, T., & Hurwitz, B. (1999). Narrative based medicine: Why study narrative? *BMJ, 318,* 48–50.

Grossard, C., Grynspan, O., Serret, S., Jouen, A.-L., Bailly, K., & Cohen, C. (2017). Serious games to teach social interactions and emotions to individuals with autism spectrum disorders (ASD). *Computers & Education, 113,* 195–211.

Hassabis, D., & Maguire, E. A. (2007). Deconstructing episodic memory with construction. *Trends in Cognitive Sciences, 11*(7), 299–306.

Heidegger, M. (1950/1994). *Holzwege* (7th ed.). Frankfurt-am-Main: Vittorio Klostermann.

Holden, M. P., Curby, K. M., Newcombe, N. S., & Shipley, T. F. (2010). A category adjustment approach to memory for spatial location in natural scenes. *Journal of Experimental Psychology: Learning, Memory, and Cognition, 36*(3), 590–604.

Hutcheson, A. T., & Wedell, D. H. (2009). Moderating the route angularity effect in a virtual environment: Support for a dual memory representation. *Memory & Cognition, 37*(4), 514–521.

James, H. (1903/2008). *The ambassadors.* London: Penguin Classics.

Lakoff, G., & Johnson, M. (1999). *Philosophy in the flesh: The embodied mind and its challenge to Western thought.* New York: Basic Books.

Levine, M., Jankovic, I. N., & Palij, M. (1982). Principles of spatial problem solving. *Journal of Experimental Psychology: General, 111,* 157–175.

Lucas, G. (1977–2005). *Star Wars* (Episodes I-VI) [Films]. Los Angeles, CA: 20th Century Fox.

Mausbach, B. T., Harvey, P. D., Goldman, S. R., Jeste, D. V., & Patterson, T. L. (2007). Development of a brief scale of everyday functioning in persons with serious mental illness. *Schizophrenia Bulletin, 33*(6), 1364–1372.

Meilinger, T., Berthoz, A., & Wiener, J. M. (2011). The integration of spatial information across different viewpoints. *Memory & Cognition, 39,* 1042–1054.

Michaelian, K. (2016). *Mental time travel: Episodic memory and our knowledge of the personal past.* Cambridge: MIT Press.

Michaelian, K., Klein, S. B., & Szpunar, K. K. (Eds.). (2016). *Seeing the future: Theoretical perspectives on future-oriented mental time travel.* New York: Oxford University Press.

Nardini, M., Thomas, R. L., Knowland, V. C. P., Braddick, O. J., & Atkinson, J. (2009). A viewpoint-independent process for spatial reorientation. *Cognition, 112,* 241–248.

Newman, E. L., Caplan, J. B., Kirschen, M. P., Korolev, I. O., Sekuler, R., & Kahana, M. J. (2007). Learning your way around town: How virtual taxi-cab drivers learn to use both layout and landmark information. *Cognition, 104,* 231–253.

Park, K., Lee, S., Yang, J., & Song, T. (2019, February 4). A systematic review and meta-analysis on the effect of reminiscence therapy for people with dementia. *International Psychogeriatrics.* Retrieved February 24, 2019, from https://doi.org/10.1017/S1041610218002168.

Plagnol, A. (2003). Dilatation de l'espace et envol maniaque. *Annales Médico-Psychologiques, 161,* 164–167.

Plagnol, A. (2004). *Espaces de représentation: Théorie élémentaire et psycho-pathologie* [Representational spaces: Elements and psychopathology]. Paris: Editions du CNRS.

Plagnol, A. (2007). Psychologie, épistémologie et théorie de la représenta-tion: fondation analogique et données séminales. *Psychologie Française, 52,* 327–339.

Plagnol, A. (in press). *Principes de navigation dans les mondes possibles* [Principles of navigation in possible worlds]. Garches, France: Terra Cotta.

Plagnol, A., Oïta, M., Montreuil, M., Granger, B., & Lubart, T. (2003). La fragmentation de l'espace de représentation dans les schizophrénies. *L'Encéphale, XXIX,* 401–411.

Plato. (≈364BC/1993). *Philebus* (D. Frede, Trans.). Indianapolis, In: Hackett.

Plato. (≈366BC/1999). *Statesman* (C. Rowe, Trans.). Indianapolis, In: Hackett.

Plato. (≈385BC/1977). *Phaedo* (G. M. A. Grube, Trans.). Indianapolis, In: Hackett.

Potts, G. R., & Peterson, S. B. (1985). Incorporation versus compartmen-talization in memory for discourse. *Journal of Memory and Language, 24,* 107–118.

Raisig, S., Welke, T., Hagendorf, H., & van der Meer, E. (2009). Insights into knowledge representation: The influence of amodal and perceptual var-iables on event knowledge retrieval from memory. *Cognitive Science, 33,* 1252–1266.

Reder, L. M., & Ross, B. H. (1983). Integrated knowledge in different tasks: The role of retrieval strategy on fan effects. *Journal of Experimental Psychology: Learning, Memory, and Cognition, 9,* 55–72.

Roberts, G. A. (2000). Narrative and severe mental illness: What place do stories have in an evidenced-based world? *Advances in Psychiatric Treatment, 6,* 432–441.

Rowling, J. K. (1997–2007). *Harry Potter* (Vol. 7). London: Bloomsbury.

Ruddle, R. A., Volkova, E., Mohler, B., & Bülthoff, H. H. (2011). The effect of landmark and body-based sensory information on route knowledge. *Memory & Cognition, 39,* 686–699.

Rumelhart, D. E. (1975). Notes on a schema for stories. In D. G. Bobrow & A. M. Collins (Eds.), *Representation and understanding: Studies in cognitive science* (pp. 211–236). New York: Academic Press.

Ruse, S. A., Harvey, P. D., Davis, V. G., Atkins, A. S., Fox, K. H., & Keefe, R. S. (2014). Virtual reality functional capacity assessment in schizophrenia: Preliminary data regarding feasibility and correlations with cognitive and functional capacity performance. *Schizophrenia Research: Cognition, 1*(1), e21–e26.

Schacter, D. L., Addis, D. R., & Buckner, R. L. (2008). Episodic simulations of future events: Concepts, data, and applications. *Annals of the New York Academy of Sciences, 1124,* 39–60.

Scott, W. (1823/2011). *Quentin durward.* London: Penguin Classics.

Siddiqui, I., Saperia, S., Fervaha, G., Da Silva, S., Jeffay, E., Zakzanis, K. K., … Foussias, G. (2018, November 22). Goal-directed planning and action impairments in schizophrenia evaluated in a virtual environment. *Schizophrenia Research*. Retrieved February 22, 2019, from https://doi.org/10.1016/j.schres.2018.10.012.

Suddendorf, T., & Corballis, M. C. (2007). The evolution of foresight: What is mental time travel, and is it unique to humans? *Behavioral and Brain Sciences, 30,* 299–351.

Szpunar, K. K. (2010). Evidence for an implicit influence of memory on future thinking. *Memory & Cognition, 38*(5), 531–540.

Thorndyke, P. W., & Hayes-Roth, B. (1982). Differences in spatial knowledge acquired from maps and navigation. *Cognitive Psychology, 14,* 560–589.

Trope, Y., & Liberman, N. (2010). Construal-level theory of psychological distance. *Psychological Review, 117*(2), 440–463.

Tulving, E. (1985). Memory and consciousness. *Canadian Psychology, 26,* 1–12.

Tulving, E. (2002). Episodic memory: From mind to brain. *Annual Review of Psychology, 53,* 1–25.

Uttal, D. H., Friedman, A., Hand, L. L., & Warren, C. (2010). Learning fine-grained and category information in navigable real-world space. *Memory & Cognition, 38*(8), 1026–1040.

van Elk, M., van Schie, H. T., & Bekkering, H. (2009). Short-term action intentions overrule long-term semantic knowledge. *Cognition, 111,* 72–83.

Waller, D., Friedman, A., Hodgson, E., & Greenauer, N. (2009). Learning scenes from multiples views: Novel views can be recognized more efficiently than learned views. *Memory & Cognition, 37*(1), 90–99.

Winnicott, D. W. (1971/2005). *Playing and reality.* London and New York: Routledge.

Zawadzki, J. A., Girard, T. A., Foussias, G., Rodrigues, A., Siddiqui, I., Lerch, J. P., ... Wong, A. H. C. (2013, November 26). Simulating real world functioning in schizophrenia using a naturalistic city environment and single-trial, goal-directed navigation. *Frontiers in Behavioral Neuroscience.* Retrieved February 22, 2019, from https://doi.org/10.3389/fnbeh.2013.00180.

Zhang, X., Xiao, H., & Chen, Y. (2017). Effect of life review on mental health and well-being among cancer patients: A systematic review. *International Journal of Nursing Studies, 74,* 138–148.

Zwaan, R. A., & Radvansky, G. A. (1998). Situation models in language comprehension and memory. *Psychological Bulletin, 123,* 162–185.

11

High-Level Navigation

1   Introduction

Some forms of mental travel can be described as "high level" navigation, because they involve the deepest dimensions of our inner worlds and the most complex refinement of our mental life. Their clinical interest is clear in that they are constantly used in psychological care, as we will see, even if their scientific bases are far from being elucidated.

We will first study what can be achieved by taking better account of the inner worlds for a type of navigation that constitutes the very heart of social life, namely "epistemic" navigation, i.e. the encounter with the inner world of oneself or of others. We will then make a brief incursion into three fields of the most valued human activities: aesthetics, science and spirituality. Not only do these fields embrace some striking achievements of the human mind, but exploring their scope from the perspective of the inner worlds is proving very fruitful for understanding client issues and therapy, so that by closing this book, we would like to give a foretaste of the exciting prospects that are opening up for research in cognitive psychodynamics.

© The Author(s) 2019
T. Ward and A. Plagnol, *Cognitive Psychodynamics as an Integrative Framework in Counselling Psychology and Psychotherapy*,
https://doi.org/10.1007/978-3-030-25823-8_11

2   Epistemic Navigation

To represent the world of others has obviously been decisive for the evolution of the human species (Brüne & Brüne-Cohrs, 2006), this capacity being the source of all cooperation (or deception!). The stages of child development directly reflect its progressive maturation, autistic disorders showing *a contrario* the major difficulties of a human being which can be encountered when meeting the world of others (Baron-Cohen, 2000). In fact, everyone has prodigious resources in epistemic navigation, even if they are unaware of it, to such an extent that the origin of certain mental disorders is sometimes less related to their defect than to their excess—hyperemotionality in social relations has been mentioned in many disorders including certain forms of autism.[1]

2.1   Simulation and Inner Worlds

In cognitive science, epistemic travel is usually approached from the angle of the attribution of mental states to others (beliefs, emotions, values, desires…), considered today through various conceptual frameworks such as *mind reading* (e.g. Goldman, 2006) or *theory of mind* (e.g. Brüne & Brüne-Cohrs, 2006), commonly integrated into the broader framework of *social cognition* (e.g. Fiske & Taylor, 2017). However, the attribution of mental states has not always been considered as a true encounter with the world of others. The attribution of a belief or desire has long been characterized as a "propositional attitude", which facilitated logical formalization, but was sometimes far removed from the person's real lived world. Studies in philosophy or experimental psychology are often still based only on elementary examples such as "Bill desires a glass of apple juice", far from the real social life in its richest aspects, for example, as it appears in a romantic encounter.

The framework of simulation theory is an important step forward in bringing us closer to the inner world of others. According to the central idea of this theory, to truly understand a mental state, it is necessary to experience it oneself in a simulation mode. Goldman (2006) and

---

[1]See, for example, the (debated) "Intense World Theory" (Markram & Markram, 2010).

Hurley (2008) have thus proposed sophisticated models of the emergence of mind reading from simulation. Oosterwijk et al. (2012) state that simulation "allows us to grasp mental states from inside out" (p. 98); Baumeister and Masicampo (2010) argue that through simulation we see people "empathically intuiting the perspectives and mental states" (p. 945); finally, simulation would enable us to develop a rich intersubjectivity (Decety & Grèzes, 2006). However, considering the simulation capability within the more general framework of epistemic navigation makes it possible to enrich its scope, particularly from a clinical perspective such as the one that the cognitive-psychodynamic approach aims to develop.

2.1.1 Complex Nesting of Worlds

The attribution of beliefs, values and desires, to its full extent, requires complex nesting of worlds of different types:

- The attribution of a belief presupposes the representation of an inner world: believing something is representing something in one's world. For example, if Tom believes that the Earth is flat, he is evolving in a world where the Earth is flat; if Sally believes that the Earth is round and Sally represents this belief of Tom, by actually deploying its content, Sally must specify in her mental space a "compartment" representing Tom's world, partly different from her own.
- An empathic emotional attribution involves the "deployment" of the emotion itself (and not simply its verbal identification from signs manifesting it). For example, authentically attributing happiness to another person means partially "unfolding" his or her happy experience as such. A full emotional attribution is therefore based on a simulation (e.g., Baumeister & Masicampo, 2010; Decety & Grèzes, 2006; Goldman, 2006; Shanton & Goldman, 2010), provided that such a simulation is conceived as the mental unfolding of a scenario, i.e. the dynamic deployment of a fragment of the world attributed to the subject concerned, with the correlative variations in tension on this fragment (passage from one emotional state to another), accompanied by the necessary epistemic markers/pointers (i.e. symbols indicating that this world is the world of this or that subject, possibly oneself—see Chapter 9, Sect. 3.3).

- Emotions are often associated with memories (e.g. regret) or expectations (e.g. hope), hence, the need for time markers entangled with epistemic markers.
- A desire implies a state that is not realized but is imaginary, what we will call a *desirable intuition* (see Plagnol, 2004, in press-a). The attribution of a desire to a subject therefore presupposes a multi-level nesting of worlds: we must represent the world of the one to whom we attribute the desire and, within this world, a desirable intuition, differentiated from the real situation. Moreover, to truly represent the desire of the other as a driving force, and to understand why he or she undertakes such-and-such an action, it is necessary to understand *what makes the desired intuition desirable*, so it is necessary to be able to simulate emotions corresponding to the tension of the desire and its resolution, whilst attributing them to the other. This implies representing evolutions of the other's inner world, with positive or negative emotions triggered by the filling or not of desirable intuitions.

> The attribution of desirable intuitions allows us to account for the search for goals and to explain the actions of others. However, without the reproduction of emotions by simulating scenarios, with the attribution of these emotions to the subject concerned, a desirable intuition could not itself be explained. We can even consider that the emergence of desire depends on such simulations: the simulation of a pleasure generally produces a pleasure anticipating the one that would be associated with its actual realization (Baumeister & Masicampo, 2010, p. 959; Plagnol 2004, in press-a). For example, if I want a chocolate cake so much so that I take action towards such a cake, it is because I am able to imagine the scenario of the cake's intake and to already experience partially the pleasure associated with this intake (see also Bagozzi, Baumgarten, & Pieters [1998] and the section on the role of emotion in decision making in Chapter 2, Sect. 7).
>
> It has been noted that the prefrontal reward circuit can induce by simulation a positive pre-goal attainment affect—for example, the simulation of a reward associated with the perception of another's smile induces pleasure (Niedenthal, Mermillod, Maringer, & Hess, 2010, p. 422).[2]

---

[2]In general, according to Lindquist, Wagner, Kober, Bliss-Moreau, and Barett (2012), "studies in which people are asked to imagine an emotional scenario probably create real experiences (as anyone knows who has become immersed in a mental reverie)" (p. 141).

In general, to attribute mental states, we engage in complex explorations by simulation of the inner worlds of others (or ourselves), using sets of modal, temporal and epistemic pointers (see Chapter 9, Sect. 3.3), and the associated emotional valences are crucial to account for these explorations.

2.1.2 Intersubjectivity

The development of an authentic intersubjectivity requires particularly refined capabilities for simulating internal worlds.

- To be truly in an intersubjective relationship, it is necessary not only to attribute desirable intuitions with emotions to oneself and to others, but also to *represent the differences* between these internal worlds, in particular the differences in values guiding possible actions. Such intersubjective differences are here again associated with imaginary complex explorations for which the simulation capacity takes its full scope.

- Finally, in the deepest intersubjective relationship, a subject must not only represent the inner world of another, but the way in which he/she is himself/herself represented in this inner other's world, so that desirable non-dual intuitions are attributed to himself/herself and to the other about what each desires of the other. The other is thus "recognized" in his/her desire different from the desire that the subject recognizes for himself/herself; hence, the dynamics of mutual representations that feed each other open up a potentially infinite space with ever new horizons.

> The encounter with another human being is decisive for the deepening of the inner world because this other one him/herself offers a new inner world, a dynamic world itself, with emotions and desires capable of modulating according to those of the other, or even moulding itself on them. Such a process of mutual co-representation, by constantly opening up new directions, offers unlimited possibilities for expansion.
>
> Any human encounter can in principle generate such an experience of enriching one's inner world by meeting the inner world of the other, as can be discovered when one has the chance to practice psychotherapy

or to encounter other humans for whom one is first unaware of such an infinite possibility of interaction (e.g. severe mental disability).

However, a romantic encounter is the privileged opportunity for such an experience, as poets have sung since antiquity. Indeed, in such a case, the intersubjective difference, based on the sensual power of sexuality, can generate an *erotic helix*, i.e. a couple of two desirable reciprocal intuitions that feed on each other, resulting in an infinite expansion of the two inner worlds. In the *Phaedrus* (≈375BC/1995), Plato speaks of a flow and counter-flow of *himeros* ("desire") that carries lovers towards *hyperouranos*—the beyond of the world....[3]

What are the signs of erotic helix formation? The most frequent manifestation of this is the exchange of glances,[4] but vision is not necessary: the timbre of the voices, the rhythm of the breaths or the skin contact, are very powerful revealing factors of an erotic helix, as blind people well know (Plagnol, in press-b).

2.2   Contributions of Cognitive Science

Epistemic navigation therefore requires sophisticated use of pointers to ensure the representation of beliefs, values and desires. However, this navigation is based on the same basic tools as spatial navigation or fictional navigation. We have already mentioned the epistemic worlds about fictional navigation, a major interest of which is the discovery of the inner worlds of characters (see Chapter 10, Sect. 3.2). Let us give some examples of the interest of an approach of the inner worlds in the light of the development of cognitive science for the study of *real* social interactions:

- The analysis of functional compartmentalization (see Chapter 9, Sect. 3.3) enables us to model the relationships between inner worlds attributed to different people (e.g. oneself and one's object of love,

---

[3]Plato, *Phaedrus* (247c, 251c, 255c).

[4]Eye contact is sufficient to trigger an empathic simulation of what the others' face express, for example, the meaning of his/her smiles, and the activation of the brain circuit "of the reward" may be directly linked to this intimate connection (Niedenthal et al., 2010).

one's therapist, etc.): boundaries, "waterproofness"/porosity, complementarity... It becomes possible to specify the degrees of separation between inner worlds, to assess the degree of fluidity of exchanges between subjective spaces and to refine notions frequently used in clinical care to characterize the proximity/mental distance between two subjects (e.g. "fusion", "mirror relationship"...).

- The decoding of the inner world of another person, so important in human relations, can benefit from a more systematic analysis of the symbolic structures that organize his/her representational space.[5] Understanding a human being's behaviour in family, social and professional contexts, is in fact based on the discovery of such symbolic structures, in particular his/her schemas—the "highways" of his/her inner world—so important to identify in social relationships, and sometimes so difficult to grasp, for example, in adolescence with regard to romantic relationships. Getting to know someone means in particular developing a network of landmarks and anchor points (that makes it easier to find one's way in his/her world).[6]

- The intimate exploration of a subject's psychological experience can be deepened if we have precise tools to describe, within his/her internal world itself, the non-actual worlds in which everyone walks daily: mind-wandering, dreaming, imagination, fantasy life, complex emotions entangled in temporal projections such as remorse or hope, desirable intuitions...

- A better consideration of globalization and focusing processes can enrich the exploration of social interactions.[7] Indeed, without realizing it, when we think about another person, we make rapid changes in scale: we use both general views of his/her inner world, for example, when we attribute this or that personality trait to him/her, and precise focalizations, for example, when we imagine his/her behaviour in this or that situation or when we project the details of an encounter. The importance of globalization/focusing phenomena

---

[5]See the definition of symbolic structures in Chapter 9, Sect. 2.3.
[6]See the notions of landmark and anchor point in Chapter 10, Sects. 2.1.1 and 2.2.
[7]See the notions of globalization and focusing in Chapter 10, Sects. 2.1.1 and 2.2.

is prominent in some attribution errors (e.g. the role of globalizing patterns in depression according to Beck's cognitive approach Beck, Rush, Shaw, & Emery, 1989). During a psychotherapeutic relationship, as during a romantic relationship, we often alternate between a synthetic vision of the other and the precise targeting of a situation that involves him/her.

2.3   Epistemic Navigation in Therapy: From Fiction to Real World

Epistemic travel is at the heart of many therapeutic techniques targeting social cognition, for example, in schizophrenia (Kurz & Richardson, 2012; Penn, Roberts, Combs, & Sterne, 2007; Peyroux & Franck, 2014; Roder, Mueller, & Schmidt, 2011). Cognitive remediation, which focuses in particular on social cognition, is now applied to numerous conditions: depression, bipolar mood extremes, personality issues and eating disturbance… (Frank, 2018; Kim et al., 2018). Such therapeutic techniques could be grounded on a more solid scientific basis and be enriched by a better understanding of the inner worlds, in particular to fill the gap between virtual worlds used in simulation techniques and real life.

Indeed, cognitive remediation techniques often are based on fictional navigation and epistemic navigation, especially on role-playing. The combination of these two types of mental navigation allows exercises of varying degrees, gradually approaching complex real-life situations. However, as any therapist knows, many of a client's problems can also be linked to difficulties to take the decisive step from virtual life to real life. Today, addictions to virtual life are on the rise, with the Internet offering unlimited ways to take refuge in such a life (Zajac, Ginley, Chang, & Petry, 2017).

However, therapy must stay focused on real life. The difference between functional capacity and real-world functioning is an important issue in the care of mental conditions such as schizophrenia (Bowie, Reichenberg, Patterson, Heaton, & Harvey, 2006; Plagnol & Pachoud, 2016). In fact, a critical problem in the field of social cognitive training is to reduce the "life-lab gap" (Fiszdon & Reddy, 2012; Franck, 2018; Henderson, 2013), in particular to extend the benefits obtained with targeted simulation exercises to real life. Work on epistemic navigation focused on real situations can help to "get back to earth" (Binswanger, 1958/1989[8]), and a rigorous analysis of the client's inner world makes it possible to specify the anchor points between the imaginary and the real, to target strategic situations and to prepare test encounters, for example, with regard to professional environment or romantic relationships. In a word, *better helping someone to meet the (outer) real world implies relying on his/her inner world.*

Finally, the therapeutic relationship offers a valuable paradigm for better understanding one's epistemic navigation abilities in the light of the exploration of one's inner world and that of others, and for developing an in-depth metacognition of it. In particular, the importance of anchor points in reality manifests itself in the therapeutic context, for example, to set limits to an overflowing fantasy, whether that of the client or the therapist—which therapist has not once hit themselves on the wall of reality after having fantasized about a client by ignoring both the client's inner world and their own world? As we mentioned in the introduction of this book, according to Carl Rogers' fundamental ideas, the success of a therapy is a direct reflection of the therapist's ability to meet the client's world as such—that is, the therapist's empathy—which includes the lucid discovery of their own inner world.

3   Aesthetic Navigation

Aesthetic experience is often presented as the encounter of a world opened through an artwork. For example, we talk about the *Iliad's* world, the *Magic Flute's* world... We also talk about the world of Homer, Mozart, etc. Indeed, the notion of world (or universe) has long been introduced in aesthetics (e.g. Goodman, 1978; Walton, 1990): to be sensitive to a work of art would be to meet a world.

---

[8]See Chapter 10, Sect. 2.

However, for an aesthetic experience to occur, the artwork must resonate with the inner world of the viewer/listener. The aesthetic encounter is in fact an interaction between two worlds, the world of a subject and the world opened by the artwork; beyond the world of the artwork, the world of the subject interacts with the world of the artist, but also the social and cultural world in which the artist is immersed (the world of ancient Greece, the eighteenth century's world, etc.).

The viewer/listener of a work is not a neutral receiver: his/her representational space, as constituted by his/her memory, structures the sensory impact of the work. The aesthetic experience actually engages the symbolic web of the viewer/listener. Thus, to appreciate a work of art, it is useful to know its historical context, the artist's biography, the artist's intention,[9] etc. In other words, access to the deepest dimensions of the world of the artwork is based on *symbolic structures* that the subject must have in his/her memory or that he must acquire.[10]

When someone encounters a work of art, his/her symbolic structures to culturally "decode" it are activated (if available), but when a powerful aesthetic effect occurs, more personal symbolic fragments are also activated by association. Multiple regions of the inner world are revived, psychological tension increases, images are projected into the window of presence, intuitions open new horizons (Plagnol, 2004, in press-a). This process can be repeated, supported by contemplation and/or listening to the work: new symbolic structures are activated, new resonances are induced in the symbolic web, new images emerge, etc. During a major aesthetic shock, a chain reaction occurs, so intense that it sometimes produces confounding effects such as the famous Stendhal syndrome (Bamforth, 2010). During this dialogue with the world of the work, an unlimited extension of the inner world can occur.

---

[9]For example, to understand that Andy Warhol's Brillo soapboxes are works of art, it is necessary to know about artistic design stance (Bullot & Reber, 2013, pp. 124–125 and p. 132).

[10]However, the genius of the artist also lies in his/her success in embodying a world in a work by evoking a resonance with universal symbolic structures already present in all minds. For example, according to Abbot Suger, father of the French Gothic cathedrals, the works that adorn the basilica of Saint-Denis (France) aim first and foremost to elevate the lay people into the spiritual spheres— even if the profound meaning of these works is only accessible to the most subtle clerics who alone have the symbolic structures to access this profound meaning (see Baschet, 2006, Chapter 6).

Artistic creation itself can be considered as a dialogue within the artist's inner world: the artist reveals in himself/herself the world of the artwork—the metaphor of *gestation* is frequent to evoke the creative process (e.g. Crispi, 2015). From a first mental image, or rather a first insight, resonances in the inner world occur, reactivating symbolic fragments, which themselves generate new images, new intuitions, until the new world that is gradually revealed is expressed in the production of a sensitive object: painting, sculpture, poetry… A work of art is in fact the metaphor of an intimate part of the artist's universe and opens for itself a new world, both for the artist and for those who receive it.

Given this fertility of aesthetic navigation—a true dialogue between worlds—artistic practice has long been used in the field of psychotherapy, particularly in institutions, to the point of becoming a discipline in its own right (*art therapy*). Let us highlight some aspects of aesthetic navigation that are particularly valuable for the psychological support of a person and can find a privileged place in a global cognitive psychodynamics:

- The encounter of an artwork, i.e. its psychological reception, with the opening on its world and on the social and cultural worlds it condenses, is a powerful opportunity for the client to reopen his own inner world (whilst a psychological disorder implies a certain confinement).
- Receptivity also implies the client's discovery of his/her own inner world: resonances in subjective space, mobilization of symbolic structures and images that emerge from them reveal to the subject some resources in him/herself of which he/she was not aware.
- When the client becomes a creator himself/herself, for example, by painting or performing a piece of music, he/she can directly explore his/her inner world, express its deep tensions, feel the pleasure of artistic production, whilst assimilating the techniques of construction, coherence and pruning that enable to achieve a consummate work.
- Finally, artistic activity offers a wonderful opportunity for exchange with others, for example, other clients or therapists, again a source, through the diversity of views on a work of art, to discover without danger the unlimited variety of inner worlds.

4   Scientific Navigation

Science, often considered as a paragon of austerity, does not exclude navigation in possible worlds, quite the contrary: our epistemic limits force us to build extensions of the perceived world and to consider alternatives to account for reality.

- The construction of possible alternatives is already the basis of our reasoning capacities.

According to Johnson-Laird's influential theory of mental models (Johnson-Laird, 1983, 2006; Johnson-Laird & Byrne, 1991), human subjects reason by developing models representing possible alternatives. This theory has been applied to various types of logical reasoning: propositional, modal, conditional, deontic and relational... (Goodwin & Johnson-Laird, 2005, 2008; Johnson-Laird & Byrne, 2002; Mackiewicz & Johnson-Laird, 2012). The experiments carried out in this framework confirm the human capacity to represent multiple alternatives during reasoning, whilst demonstrating the impact on this capacity of the limits of working memory, hence, the need for "navigation" between the models of alternatives.

Similarly, counterfactual reasoning, probability estimation, calculation of utilities or costs, decision theory with prioritisation of action, etc., require the construction of alternatives to reality with compartmentalizing between them (e.g. Barrouillet, Gauffroy, & Lecas, 2008; Busemeyer, Pothos, Franco, & Trueblood, 2011; Byrne, 2007; Dixon & Byrne, 2011; Evans, 2007; Fennell & Baddeley, 2012; Fugard, Pfeifer, Mayerhofer, & Kleiter, 2011; Kahneman & Tversky, 1982; Koehler & James, 2009; Kurzban, Duckworth, Kable, & Myers, 2013; Lombrozo, 2007; Oaksford & Chater, 2009; Sims, Neth, Jacobs, & Gray, 2013).

- Moreover, a large part of scientific activity is related to the construction of a world. Indeed, knowing a domain of reality means reconstructing the most appropriate world to integrate available data, or even future data (prediction). For example, in astronomy, observations of the sky are unified to reconstruct part of the cosmos; in criminal science, clues are collected to reconstruct a crime scenario; in palaeontology, fossils are analysed and compared to reconstruct the lives of our distant ancestors, etc. It is worth noting that the diagnostic approach in modern medicine, from the Canadian Joseph Bell (1837–1911) and the Scottish William Osler (1849–1919) to today's evidence-based practice, is based on the reconstruction of a disease from symptoms/data/evidence (Amad et al., 2018).

- Scientific experiments provide new data to extend the known world (Plagnol, 2007). Indeed, science is not the insipid validation of a closed space but the exploration of *terra incognita*, and imagination is as necessary as logical rigour for the expression of scientific genius (Holton, 1998).

- Finally, when new data cannot be integrated into the accepted version of the world, this requires a paradigm shift (Kuhn, 1970), i.e. the construction of a new world. Such data can be described as "traumatic" because they generate powerful defences, as evidenced by the fate of the Prisoner of Plato's Cave,[11] or Galileo's misadventures with the Roman Church, in the same way that a traumatic event cannot be integrated into a subjective inner world and triggers dissociative defences (see Chapter 7).

The scientific navigation model, combining rigour and imagination for the exploration of the real world, can feed therapeutic work on the inner world. However, to our knowledge, this model has not been widely used, with the notable exception of the cognitive-behavioural framework, which invites the client to draw inspiration from the scientific approach to test the implicit hypotheses generated by his/her internal schemas (e.g. at the origin of automatic thoughts leading to a pessimistic conception of the world (Beck et al., 1989). Moreover, some aspects of the psychoanalytical method as practiced by Freud may be similar to the reconstruction of a scenario/world based on clues such as dreams, missed acts, etc.[12]

Scientific navigation can enrich psychotherapeutic work in many ways. Indeed, scientific navigation offers a fertile model for:

---

[11]Plato (≈375BC/1992), *Republic, VII*, 514a–519e.

[12]See, for example, *Delusions and Dreams in Jensen's Gradiva* (Freud, 1907/1959).

- more finely testing clients' implicit assumptions, by inviting them to consider systematic variations of scenarios constructed from their experiences and by showing that such scenarios reflect their inner world and its symbolic structures;
- highlight the multiple resources of access to the imagination, which can be valuable in subjects haunted by fear of being irrational and/or who defend themselves by severe means against their fantasies, for example, obsessive-compulsive subjects;
- build unified worlds, combining intuition and reasoning, exploration and rigorous control, creativity and concern for coherence, crossing known borders and anchoring in the real world through relevant experimental probes.
- reconstruct a story from scraps of memory, just as a scientist reconstructs a scenario from a few data—for example, the rise and fall of the Roman Empire from lead rates in the arctic ice layers (McConnell et al., 2018). In particular, the scientific need to reconfigure the known world when it is hit by "traumatic" data (paradigm shift) can serve as a neutral model for integrating a traumatic event into an inner world when its foundations are shaken, eventually opening up to richer extensions once the ordeal is overcome.

5   Spiritual Navigation

The importance of spiritual life in care situations is increasingly recognized (e.g. Puchalski, 2004; Hordern, 2016; Moreira-Almeida, Sharma, Janse van Resburg, Verhagen, & Cook, 2016). It has been shown in many contexts that support for religious beliefs can help clients overcome suffering that would otherwise be unbearable: palliative care situations (Richardson, 2014), bereavement of a loved one (Lomas, Timmins, Harley, & Mates, 2004; Walsh, King, Jones, Tookman, & Blizard, 2002), severe trauma (see Chapter 7, Sect. 4.4)… Care that is truly centred on people—both caretakers and carers—cannot ignore this aspect of life that many people consider to be the basis of their values and their existence (e.g. Fulford, Peile, & Carroll, 2012).

The spiritual life is often conceived as an effort to free oneself from the contingencies of the ordinary world and to encounter a form of deeper presence, or even another world situated in another order of reality. The seminal writings of the great religions abound in metaphors borrowed from the field of travel, starting with the need to "convert" (redirect oneself towards the true good), "get on the way", "set off on a journey". Ancient mythologies already considered death as a migration of the soul from one world to another. Poetic and pictorial representations sometimes wonderfully illustrate how a spiritual quest is always a spiritual travel–let us think, for example, of the *Divine Comedy* and the initiation that leads Dante, accompanied by Virgil and then by Beatrice, from the circles of Hell to Paradise through Purgatory (Dante, ≈1307–1321/2012).

However, the spiritual quest, if it can aim at a transcendent exteriority, for example, that of a Kingdom outside the common world, is often apprehended in close correspondence with the inner world. For some mystics, the Kingdom is even to be sought in oneself: the masterpiece of Saint Teresa of Avila is entitled "The Interior Castle" (Saint Teresa of Avila, 1588/2015), whilst the Home ideal (see Chapter 7, Sect. 4.3.2) is directly transposed from the inner world to the reception within God in the Christian religion (countless references to the home of God in the Psalms and the Gospels). A similar theme is present in other great religious frameworks: let's just recall, for example, the famous poem by the Muslim mystic Djalâl ad-Dîn Rûmî, *The Guest House* (Thirteenth century/1996), which today inspires the mindfulness-based cognitive therapy [MBCT] (Segal, Williams, & Teasdale, 2013).[13]

The spiritual universe thus refers the believer back to the heart of the deepest aspects of his/her inner world (because these aspects are perceived as the foundations of its totality), the most extensive (because they aim at infinity and eternity) and the most interior (because they are associated with the most extreme emotions such as despair or hope).

Taking spiritual navigation into account can therefore provide the therapist with a more intimate understanding of his/her client and the

---

[13]This poem illustrates the main axis towards which all MBCT sessions tend, according to Mirabel-Sarron, Docteur, Sala, Siobud-Dorocant, and Penet (2018).

resources available to him/her—even to recognize an irreducible difference if the religious world of the client is too far away from the therapist's personal world. Whatever the difference, the therapist can rely on what is proposed in the client's spiritual horizon to help him/her overcome ordeals, soothe his/her inner world upset by illness or grief and regain hope by discovering the possibility of meaning beyond an intolerable hardship, as expressed by the great French poet Victor Hugo (1856/1911) after the death of his daughter Leopoldine:

> *Ô mon Dieu! Cette plaie a si longtemps saigné !*
> *L'angoisse dans mon âme est toujours la plus forte,*
> *Et mon cœur est soumis, mais n'est pas résigné.*[14]

As Fulford, Peile, and Carroll (2012) point out, spiritual guidance techniques have long inspired counselling, not only to support the overcoming of life's ordeals, but also to orient oneself in the forest of desires, to make a choice according to one's values, to discover new directions for life, etc. that is, in a word and to explore the unknown wealth of one's inner world. Perhaps the time has come to renew such an exploration by using the most recent tools developed in cognitive science to better deepen the infinite potential of such a world.

6   Concluding Remarks

In order to clarify the potential of the cognitive-psychodynamic approach, by confronting it with ambitious objectives, we have tried to outline some new boundaries to explore the most prized fields of human activity, from erotic life to spiritual life, including artistic and scientific life.

---

[14]"*Oh my God! This wound has bled for so long/Anguish in my soul is always the strongest/And my heart is obedient, but not resigned*" (our translation). *A Villequier* was written by Hugo on 4 September 1847, 4 years to the day after Leopoldine drowned in the Seine at the age of 19 (which Hugo learned 5 days later by reading the newspaper *Le Siècle* on his way back from Spain). This tragic and spiritual experience of the great French romantic poet can be compared to Lamartine's at the death of his daughter Julia, mentioned in Chapter 7, Sect. 4.4 (see also Plagnol, 2014).

In any case, it must be clear that the psychodynamic-cognitive approach does not propose a revolution: these fields have long been explored by multiple disciplines and many paths already cross them in a therapeutic perspective. However, from a clinical point of view, these fields are rarely addressed in a unified way due to the lack of tools fine enough to truly integrate their contribution. In particular, methods that were hitherto based on a cognitive perspective have hardly been able to exploit the richness of insights from qualitative methods, notably phenomenological and psychodynamic, to which the approach to this high-level navigation has long been reserved.

Advances in cognitive science, which ground a better understanding of the inner worlds, can now help to bring together the contributions of these different conceptual frameworks in order to better account for the full dynamics of mental life and the prodigious richness it conceals, even in the most severe conditions (which in fact always reflect this richness). An integrated framework for the study of high-level mental navigation, as proposed by the cognitive-psychodynamic approach, opens up promising new horizons for research and clinical applications.

References

Amad, A., Geoffroy, P. A., Micoulaud-Franchi, J.-A., Bensamoun, D., Benzerouk, F., Peyre, H., …, Fovet, T. (2018). L'examen clinique standardisé pour étudiants, c'est possible ! *Annales Médico-Psychologiques, 176*(9), 936–940.

Bagozzi, R. P., Baumgartner, H., & Pieters, R. (1998). Goal-directed emotions. *Cognition and Emotion, 12*(1), 1–26.

Bamforth, I. (2010). Stendhal's syndrome. *British Journal of General Practice, 60*(581), 945–946.

Baron-Cohen, S. (2000). Theory of mind and autism: A review. *International Review of Research in Mental Retardation, 23,* 169–184.

Barrouillet, P., Gauffroy, C., & Lecas, J.-F. (2008). Mental models and the suppositional account of conditionals. *Psychological Review, 115*(3), 760–772.

Baschet, J. (2006). *La civilisation féodale — De l'an mil à la colonisation de l'Amérique* [Feudal civilization—From the year 1000 to the colonization of America] (3rd ed.). Paris: Flammarion.

Baumeister, R. F., & Masicampo, E. J. (2010). Conscious thought is for facilitating social and cultural interactions: How mental simulations serve the animal-culture interface. *Psychological Review, 117*(3), 945–971.

Beck, A., Rush, A. J., Shaw, B. F., & Emery, G. (1989). *Cognitive therapy of depression.* New York: Guilford.

Binswanger, L. (1958/1989). Analyse existentielle et psychothérapie (II). In *Introduction à l'analyse existentielle* [Introduction to existential analysis] (J. Verdaux & R. Kuhn, Trans., pp. 149–157). Paris: Minuit.

Bowie, C. R., Reichenberg, A., Patterson, T. L., Heaton, R. K., & Harvey, P. D. (2006). Determinants of real-world functional performance in schizophrenia subjects: Correlations with cognition, functional capacity, and symptoms. *American Journal of Psychiatry, 163*(3), 418–425.

Brüne, M., & Brüne-Cohrs, U. (2006). Theory of mind—Evolution, ontogeny, brain mechanisms and psychopathology. *Neuroscience and Biobehavioral Reviews, 30*(4), 437–455.

Bullot, N. J., & Reber, R. (2013). The artful mind meets art history: Toward a psycho-historical framework for the science of art appreciation. *Behavioral and Brain Sciences, 36,* 123–180.

Busemeyer, J. R., Pothos, E. M., Franco, R., & Trueblood, J. S. (2011). A quantum theoretical explanation for probability judgment errors. *Psychological Review, 118,* 193–218.

Byrne, R. M. J. (2007). Précis of 'The rational imagination: How people create alternatives to reality'. *Behavioral and Brain Sciences, 30,* 439–480.

Crispi, L. (2015). *Joyce's creative process and the construction of characters in Ulysses: Becoming the Blooms.* Oxford: Oxford University Press.

Dante. (≈1307–1321/2012). *The Divine comedy: Inferno, Purgatori, Paradiso* (R. Kirkpatrick, Trans.). London: Penguin classics.

Decety, J., & Grèzes, J. (2006). The power of simulation: Imagine one's own and other's bevavior. *Brain Research, 1079*(1), 4–14.

Dixon, J. E., & Byrne, R. M. J. (2011). "If only" counterfactual thoughts about exceptional actions. *Memory & Cognition, 39,* 1317–1331.

Evans, J. St. B. T. (2007). *Hypothetical thinking: Dual processes in reasoning and judgment.* Hove: Psychology Press.

Fennell, J., & Baddeley, R. (2012). Uncertainty plus priors equals rational bias: An intuitive bayesian probability weighting function. *Psychological Review, 119*(4), 878–887.

Fiske, S. T., & Taylor, S. E. (2017). *Social cognition: From brains to culture* (3rd ed.). London: Sage.

Fiszdon, J. M., & Reddy, L. F. (2012). Review of social cognitive treatments for psychosis. *Clinical Psychology Review, 32*(8), 724–740.

Franck, N. (2018). Développements en remédiation cognitive. In A. Plagnol, B. Pachoud, & B. Granger (Eds.), *Les Nouveaux modèles de soins — une clinique au service de la personne* [New models of care: A clinical practice at the service of the person] (pp. 87–97). Montrouge, France: Doin.

Freud, S. (1907/1959). Delusions and dreams in Jensen's *Gradiva*. In J. Strachey (Ed.), *The standard edition of the complete psychological works of Sigmund Freud, Volume IX (1906–1908): Jensen's Gradiva and other works* (pp. 7–96). London: The Hogarth Press and the Institute of Psychoanalysis.

Fugard, A. J. B., Pfeifer, N., Mayerhofer, B., & Kleiter, G. D. (2011). How people interpret conditionals: Shifts towards the conditional event. *Journal of Experimental Psychology. Learning, Memory, and Cognition, 37*, 635–648.

Fulford, K. W. M. (Bill), Peile, E., & Carroll, H. (2012). Elective fertility: Think high-tech, think evidence and values! Values-based practice element 9: The Science-driven principle. In *Essential values-based practice: Clinical stories linking science with people* (pp. 151–162). Cambridge: Cambridge University Press.

Goldman, A. I. (2006). *Simulating minds: The philosophy, psychology, and neuroscience of mindreading.* Oxford: Oxford University Press.

Goodman, N. (1978). *Ways of worldmaking.* Indianapolis, IN: Hackett.

Goodwin, G. P., & Johnson-Laird, P. N. (2005). Reasoning about relations. *Psychological Review, 112*, 468–493.

Goodwin, G. P., & Johnson-Laird, P. N. (2008). Transitive and pseudo-transitive inferences. *Cognition, 108*, 320–352.

Henderson, A. R. (2013). The impact of social cognition training on recovery from psychosis. *Current Opinion in Psychiatry, 26*(5), 429–432.

Holton, G. (1998). *The scientific imagination.* Cambridge, MA: Harvard University Press.

Hordern, J. (2016). Religion and culture. *Medicine, 44*(10), 589–592.

Hugo, V. (1856/1911). A Villequier. In V. Hugo (Ed.), *Les Contemplations* [The contemplations] (pp. 254–259). Paris: Nelson. Retrieved February 28, 2019, from https://fr.wikisource.org/wiki/Les_Contemplations/À_Villequier.

Hurley, S. (2008). The shared circuit model (SCM): How control, mirroring, and simulation can enable imitation, deliberation, and mindreading. *Behavioral and Brain Sciences, 31*, 1–58.

Johnson-Laird, P. N. (1983). *Mental models: Towards a cognitive science of language, inference, and consciousness.* Cambridge: Cambridge University Press.

Johnson-Laird, P. N. (2006). *How we reason*. New York: Oxford University Press.

Johnson-Laird, P. N., & Byrne, R. M. J. (1991). *Deduction*. Hillsdale, NJ: Lawrence Erlbaum Associates.

Johnson-Laird, P. N., & Byrne, R. M. J. (2002). Conditionals: A theory of meaning, pragmatics, and inference. *Psychological Review, 109,* 646–678.

Kahneman, D., & Tversky, A. (1982). *Judgment under uncertainty: Heuristics and biases*. New York: Cambridge University Press.

Kim, E. J., Bahk, Y.-C., Oh, H., Lee W.-H., Lee, J.-S., & Choi, K.-H. (2018, October 1). Current status of cognitive remediation for psychiatric disorders: A review. *Frontiers in Psychiatry*. Retrieved February 26, 2019, from https://doi.org/10.3389/fpsyt.2018.00461.

Koehler, D. J., & James, G. (2009). Probability matching in choice under uncertainty: Intuition versus deliberation. *Cognition, 113,* 123–127.

Kuhn, T. S. (1970). *The structure of scientific revolutions* (2nd ed.). Chicago: University of Chicago Press.

Kurtz, M. M., & Richardson, C. L. (2012). Social cognitive training for schizophrenia: A meta-analytic investigation of controlled research. *Schizophrenia Bulletin, 38*(5), 1092–1104.

Kurzban, R., Duckworth, A., Kable, J. W., & Myers, J. (2013). An opportunity cost model of subjective effort and task performance. *Behavioral and Brain Sciences, 36,* 661–726.

Lindquist, K. A., Wagner, T. D., Kober, H., Bliss-Moreau, E., & Barett, L. (2012). The brain basis of emotion: A meta-analytic review. *Behavioral and Brain Sciences, 35,* 121–202.

Lomas, D., Timmins, J., Harley, B., & Mates, A. (2004). The use of pastoral and spiritual support in bereavement care. *Nursing Times, 100*(1), 34–35.

Lombrozo, T. (2007). Simplicity and probability in causal explanation. *Cognitive Psychology, 55,* 232–257.

Mackiewicz, R., & Johnson-Laird, P. N. (2012). Reasoning from connectives and relations between entities. *Memory & Cognition, 40,* 266–279.

Markram, K., & Markram, H. (2010, December 21). The intense world theory—A unifying theory of the neurobiology of autism. *Frontiers in Human Neuroscience*. Retrieved February 25, 2019, from https://doi.org/10.3389/fnhum.2010.00224.

McConnell, J. R., Wilson, A. I., Stohl, A., Arienzo, M. M., Chellman, N. J., Eckardt, S., …, Steffensen, J. P. (2018). Lead pollution recorded in Greenland ice indicates European emissions tracked plagues, wars, and imperial expansion during antiquity. *Proceedings of the National Academy of Sciences of the United States of America, 115*(22), 5726–5731.

Mirabel-Sarron, C., Docteur, A., Sala, L., Siobud-Dorocant, E., & Penet, C. (2018). *Pratiquer la thérapie de pleine conscience (MBCT) pas à pas* [Practice mindfulness therapy (MBCT) step by step]. Malakoff, France: Dunod.

Moreira-Almeida, A., Sharma, A., Janse van Resburg, B., Verhagen, P. J., & Cook, C. C. H. (2016). WPA position statement on spirituality and religion in psychiatry. *World Psychiatry, 15*(1), 87–88.

Niedenthal, P. M., Mermillod, M., Maringer, M., & Hess, U. (2010). The simulation of smiles (SIMS) model: Embodied simulation and the meaning of facial expression. *Behavioral and Brain Sciences, 33*, 417–480.

Oaksford, M., & Chater, N. (2009). Précis of 'Bayesian rationality: The probabilistic approach to human reasoning'. *Behavioral and Brain Science, 32*, 69–120.

Oosterwijk, S., Winkielman, P., Pecher, D., Zeelenberg, R., Rotteveel, M., & Fischer, A. H. (2012). Mental states inside out: Switching costs for emotional and nonemotional sentences that differ in internal and external focus. *Memory & Cognition, 40*, 93–100.

Penn, D. L., Roberts, D. L., Combs, D., & Sterne, A. (2007). Best practices: The development of the Social Cognition and Interaction Training program for schizophrenia spectrum disorders. *Psychiatric Services, 58*(4), 449–451.

Peyroux, E., & Franck, N. (2014, June 13). RC2S: A cognitive remediation program to improve social cognition in schizophrenia and related disorders. *Frontiers in Human Neuroscience*. Retrieved February 26, 2019, from https://doi.org/10.3389/fnhum.2014.00400.

Plagnol, A. (2004). *Espaces de représentation: Théorie élémentaire et psychopathologie* [Representational spaces: Elements and psychopathology]. Paris: Editions du CNRS.

Plagnol, A. (2007). Psychologie, épistémologie et théorie de la représentation: fondation analogique et données séminales. *Psychologie Française, 52*, 327–339.

Plagnol, A. (2014). Douleur, souffrance et intenable. *L'Evolution Psychiatrique, 79*(4), 798–808.

Plagnol, A. (in press-a). *Principes de navigation dans les mondes possibles* [Principles of navigation in possible worlds]. Garches, France: Terra Cotta.

Plagnol, A. (in press-b). *Bains d'hiver* [Winter baths]. Garches, France: Terra Cotta.

Plagnol, A., & Pachoud, B. (2016). Capacité fonctionnelle et fonctionnement en situation réelle. In V. Boucherat-Hue et al. (Eds.), *Handicap psychique:*

questions vives [Psychic disability: Hot issues] (pp. 193–214). Toulouse, France: Erès.

Plato. (≈375BC/1992). *Republic* (G. M. A. Grube, Trans., C. D. C. Reeve, Rev.) Indianapolis, IN: Hackett.

Plato. (≈375BC/1995). *Phaedrus* (A. Nehamas & P. Woodruff, Trans.). Indianapolis, IN: Hackett.

Puchalski, C. (2004). Spirituality in health: The role of spirituality in critical care. *Critical Care Clinics, 20*(3), 487–504.

Richarson, P. (2014). Spirituality, religion and palliative care. *Annals of Palliative Medicine, 3*(3), 150–159.

Roder, V., Mueller, D. R., & Schmidt, S. J. (2011). Effectiveness of Integrated Psychological Therapy (IPT) for schizophrenia patients: A research update. *Schizophrenia Bulletin, 37*(suppl. 2), S71–S79.

Rumi. (Thirteenth century/1996). The guest house. In Rumi (Ed.) & C. Banks & J. Moyne, (Trans.), *The essential Rumi* (p. 109). New York: HarperCollins.

Saint Teresa of Avila. (1588/2015). *The Interior Castle*. London: Aeterna Press.

Segal, Z. V., Williams, J. M. G., & Teasdale, J. D. (2013). *Mindfulness-based cognitive therapy for depression* (2nd ed.). New York: Guilford Press.

Shanton, K., & Goldman, A. (2010). Simulation theory. *Wiley Interdisciplinary Reviews: Cognitive Science, 1*(4), 527–538.

Sims, C. R., Neth, H., Jacobs, R. A., & Gray, W. D. (2013). Melioration as rational choice: Sequential decision making in uncertain environments. *Psychological Review, 120*(1), 139–154.

Walsh, K., King, M., Jones, L., Tookman, A., & Blizard, R. (2002). Spiritual beliefs may affect outcome of bereavement: Prospective study. *BMJ, 324*(7353), 1551.

Walton, K. (1990). *Mimesis as make-believe: On the foundations of the representational arts*. Cambridge, MA: Harvard University Press.

Zajac, K., Ginley, M. K., Chang, R., & Petry, N. M. (2017). Treatments for Internet gaming disorder and Internet addiction: A systematic review. *Psychology of Addictive Behaviors, 31*(8), 979–994.

12

Conclusions and Future Directions

In this book, we have surveyed some of the major strands in current psychotherapeutic thinking at the start of the twenty first century. We went on to look at the findings from neuroscience, which bear on important therapeutic themes. This started with an overview of cognitive phenomenology and the notion of a global conscious workspace, underpinned by memory representations. Other important influences on behaviour include biological drives, and the ongoing emotional tone, which accompanies our actions. We also looked briefly at the current theories of psychophysiology in terms of fear, anxiety, compulsions and depression.

In Chapter 3, we outlined an approach to human motivation, based principally on the work of Grawe (2007). This puts forward a number of suggestions for what constitutes basic psychological needs, including control, avoidance of pain and satisfactory attachment relationships. By attempting to meet these, we develop behavioural patterns, called motivational schemas. Traditional defence mechanisms can be seen as motivational schemas, as can the early maladaptive schemas put forward by Young, Klosko, & Weishaar (2003).

© The Author(s) 2019
T. Ward and A. Plagnol, *Cognitive Psychodynamics as an Integrative Framework in Counselling Psychology and Psychotherapy*,
https://doi.org/10.1007/978-3-030-25823-8_12

A further chapter was devoted to memory representation. This is an important area given the importance of what we can actively recall (explicit) and the learning which guides us but of which we are not always fully aware (implicit). It was suggested that a lot of client material in therapy consists of, on the one hand self-defining memory of pivotal events and on the other exploring recurring patterns of behaviour composed of motivational schemas.

Chapter 5 gave an outline of the process of cognitive psychodynamic therapy. This consists of creating a safe space in which clients can explore their individual narrative. Typically, these narratives will include both conscious cognitive thoughts and recollections, alongside accounts of day-to-day incidents and behaviour. The therapeutic relationship itself will be shaped by the past learning and relationship history of both the client and the therapist. It can therefore be seen that cognitive psychodynamic therapy includes influences from all the major schools of therapy. We recognize that the client's life history, which has led them to a particular point, is unique to them, and therefore, it is important to explore issues from within their frame of reference (Rogers, 1951). At the same time, we acknowledge that clients will strive to understand and find meaning in their lives, which reflects basic needs around control, orientation and self-enhancement. We see people's past learning as being crucial in determining the approach they take to everyday situations and problems, especially their relationship and attachment history. Finally, we recognize that the venue in which much of this plays out is the cognitive conscious workspace of the mind. This may become dominated by negative thoughts, with our attention focused on threats and challenges, which are perceived to be insurmountable.

We then explored in some depth how the cognitive-psychodynamic perspective can be applied to three areas of client concern, with separate chapters on depression, trauma and anxiety. In each case, we considered how the condition affects the client's inner world, and how this can be mitigated in therapy.

Finally, we went on to specify in more detail how we can conceptualize the workings of the inner world and mental navigation within this realm (Plagnol, 2004, in press). We extended this consideration into wider domains such as fiction and science. From this, we then considered higher levels of travel, meeting the inner worlds of others and spirituality.

We think that the cognitive-psychodynamic paradigm offers a very fertile plane for future research and development. To begin with, there is scope to evaluate this as an effective therapeutic approach, compared to others. There is already evidence that the cognitive stance can benefit from additional relational perspectives (Newman, Castonguay, Borkovec, Fisher, & Nordberg, 2008). We ourselves are currently carrying out work on the application of cognitive psychodynamics to depression and anxiety. We are also extending the approach to work with couples, where there is already evidence of the utility of looking at patterns of relating and past learning (Snyder, 1999; Tilden & Dattilio, 2005).

Although we have concentrated on depression, trauma and anxiety, the cognitive-psychodynamic approach could be usefully extended to other client concerns. For example, in relation to addiction, there is good evidence that past learning and experience will have shaped the client's inner world such that they may wish to numb their feelings or escape their inner world through substance use (Bojed & Nikmanesh, 2013; Kellog & Tatarsky, 2012; Plagnol, 2004; Shaghaghy, Saffarinia, Iranpoor, & Soltanynejad, 2011). Motivational interviewing (Weegmann, 2002) could be seen as one way of helping addicted clients to reshape their inner world by bringing to the fore and adding structure to their motivation to change.

In the last few chapters, we referred to ways in which the cognitive-psychodynamic approach could work with clients to explore their inner worlds in new and exciting ways. There is evidence, for example, from sport psychology (Ryan & Simons, 1982) and leadership development (Neck & Manz, 1992), that activities in the realm of the inner world are by themselves sufficient to create positive real-world change. As we suggested, such activities could be augmented by virtual reality to enhance people's inner navigation (Ward et al., 2016). Research illustrating this potential already exists, for example, in relation to anxiety (Powers & Emmelkamp, 2008) and social phobia (Klinger et al., 2005). Future research could look at ways of using virtual reality in a flexible way to reflect the unique inner world of each client.

In relation to the above directions, we believe it would be useful to establish how past implicit learning patterns can be modified or deactivated. In many cases, this may be through establishing new patterns and schemas alongside the old, so that the new more adaptive pattern will be activated in preference to the old. We believe there may be a role for artificial intelligence in helping us to establish how such learning takes place and can be modified (Ward, 2008). This could lead to new suggestions and insights, which can then be tested in the therapy room.

This book will be a success for us if, at the end of its reading, therapists are concerned to better base their practice in contemporary science, whatever their allegiance, and have discovered new means to enrich their interactions with clients.

Of course, other ways are possible than ours to build on the advances of science, other tools can be proposed, other models forged, other horizons drawn. In opening the way for a cognitive-psychodynamic approach, we may have seemed sometimes too bold—or on the contrary too timid—we may have neglected multiple fields of research as exciting as they are in carrying fruitful clinical applications, and perhaps some experts or "temple guardians" may have considered that we betrayed such or such concept of cognitive science, ignored such or such important experimental data, or distorted such or such phenomenological or psychodynamic insight.

Whatever the obvious limitations of this book, we are convinced that the themes we have tried to address will increasingly become part of the psychotherapy research landscape. Indeed, a better understanding of the inner world of a client, to help him/her reshape it by him/herself in interaction with the therapist's inner world, is at the heart of any type of therapy. Isn't it time to better ground some notions constantly used to talk about therapeutic work such as *opening a door, clearing a path, finding a horizon*? To give greater scope to empathy as the encounter with the inner world of others as if it were one's own?[1] To give a

---

[1] "Accurate empathic understanding means that the therapist is completely at home in the universe of the client [...] It is the sensing of the client's inner world of private personal meanings 'as if' it were the therapist's own, but without ever losing the 'as if' quality" (Rogers & Truax, 1967, p. 104).

precise meaning to some of the most stimulating concepts for clinical research today such as *mental travel, making-meaning, seeding procedure, post-traumatic growth*? To provide therapists and clients with a refined theory of immersion in a story or game, daydreaming and mind-wandering, imagination and romance?

In fact, beyond the care of people with psychological distress, it is a true science of exploring mental universes that seems possible to us today, at the very time that navigation on the World Wide Web offers us a fascinating model—fascinating but infinitely coarser, infinitely less flexible and sophisticated than navigation in the depths of the mental universes.

If we consider the universe of psychotherapies itself in the light of the tools we have brought in, it is possible that the rigid compartmentalization between schools mentioned in our introduction may gradually evolve into a unified landscape, marked by functional boundaries that preserve from a naïve eclecticism but do not prevent the rational integration of types of practice, the complementarity of the methods, the clarification of their levels of relevance with regard to the different dimensions of the human mind—in short, a dynamic landscape that can be contextualized in a flexible way to select such or such set of clinical tools tailored to the client's inner world to help them overcome their difficulties.

Is our cognitive-psychodynamic approach likely to provide a framework to support such an evolution? We are aware of the huge work that remains to be done to justify such an ambition more firmly, both for the theoretical foundation of this approach and for its clinical validation, *a fortiori* for the exploration of fields such as those we have outlined in the last chapters of this book. But such broad perspectives of research are already for us precious fruits, as they may be the most stimulating promises of future harvests. May we have opened up desirable directions for better pioneering the worlds of human beings, their amazing capacities of mental navigation, their prodigious resources to face new worlds.

Would this finally be another way of rediscovering Carl Rogers' fundamental intuitions? The potential of each individual—a potential that psychological distress sometimes hinders but also reveals—is the expression of an infinitely rich inner world, and the exploration of this world is a key condition for the actualization of such a potential. We will be happy if this book facilitates a few small steps to deepen this intuition that supports our fundamental trust in the future of the ideas outlined here.

References

Bojed, F. B., & Nikmanesh, Z. (2013). Role of early maladaptive schemas on addiction potential in youth. *International Journal of High Risk Behaviors & Addiction, 2*(2), 72–83.

Grawe, K. (2007). *Neuropsychotherapy*. London: Psychology Press.

Kellogg, S. H., & Tatarsky, A. (2012). Re-envisioning addiction treatment: A six-point plan. *Alcoholism Treatment Quarterly, 30*(1), 109–128.

Klinger, E., Bouchard, S., Légeron, P., Roy, S., Lauer, F., Chemin, I., & Nugues, P. (2005). Virtual reality therapy versus cognitive behavior therapy for social phobia: A preliminary controlled study. *Cyberpsychology & Behavior, 8*(1), 76–88.

Neck, C. P., & Manz, C. C. (1992). Thought self-leadership: The influence of self-talk and mental imagery on performance. *Journal of Organizational Behavior, 13*(7), 681–699.

Newman, M. G., Castonguay, L. G., Borkovec, T. D., Fisher, A. J., & Nordberg, S. S. (2008). An open trial of integrative therapy for generalized anxiety disorder. *Psychotherapy: Theory, Research, Practice, Training, 45*(2), 135–148.

Plagnol, A. (2004). *Espaces de représentation: Théorie élémentaire et psychopathologie [Representational spaces: Elements and psychopathology]*. Paris: Editions du CNRS.

Plagnol, A. (in press). *Principes de navigation dans les mondes possibles [Principles of navigation in possible worlds]*. Garches, France: Terra Cotta.

Powers, M. B., & Emmelkamp, P. M. (2008). Virtual reality exposure therapy for anxiety disorders: A meta-analysis. *Journal of Anxiety Disorders, 22*(3), 561–569.

Rogers, C. R. (1951). *Client centred therapy*. London: Constable.

Rogers, C. R., & Truax, C. B. (1967). The therapeutic conditions antecedent to change: A theoretical view. In C. R. Rogers, E. T. Gendlin, D. J. Kiesler, & C. B. Truax (Eds.), *The therapeutic relationships and its impact: A study of psychotherapy with schizophrenics* (pp. 97–108). Madison, WI: University of Wisconsin Press.

Ryan, E. D., & Simons, J. (1982). Efficacy of mental imagery in enhancing mental rehearsal of motor skills. *Journal of Sport Psychology, 4*(1), 41–51.

Shaghaghy, F., Saffarinia, M., Iranpoor, M., & Soltanynejad, A. (2011). The relationship of early maladaptive schemas, attributional styles and learned helplessness among addicted and non-addicted men. *Addiction & Health, 3*(1–2), 45–58.

Snyder, D. K. (1999). Affective reconstruction in the context of a pluralistic approach to couple therapy. *Clinical Psychology: Science and Practice, 6*(4), 348–365.

Tilden, T., & Dattilio, F. M. (2005). Vulnerability schemas of individuals in couples relationships: A cognitive perspective. *Contemporary Family Therapy, 27*(2), 139–162.

Ward, T. (2008). Are connectionist models useful in counselling psychology? *Counselling Psychology Review, 23,* 97–102.

Ward, T., Falconer, L., Frutos-Perez, M., Williams, B., Johns, J., & Harold, S. (2016). Using virtual online simulations in Second Life® to engage undergraduate psychology students with employability issues. *British Journal of Educational Technology, 47*(5), 918–931.

Weegmann, M. (2002). Motivational interviewing and addiction-A psychodynamic appreciation. *Psychodynamic Practice, 8*(2), 179–195.

Young, J. E., Klosko, J. S., & Weishaar, M. E. (2003). *Schema therapy: A practitioner's guide.* New York: Guilford Press.

Index

© The Editor(s) (if applicable) and The Author(s) 2019
T. Ward and A. Plagnol, *Cognitive Psychodynamics as an Integrative
Framework in Counselling Psychology and Psychotherapy*,
https://doi.org/10.1007/978-3-030-25823-8

The manufacturer's authorised representative in the EU is Springer
Nature Customer Service Centre GmbH, Europaplatz 3, 69115 Heidelberg,
Germany. If you have any concerns regarding our products, please
contact ProductSafety@springernature.com

Printed and bound by CPI Group (UK) Ltd, Croydon, CR0 4YY
29/04/2026
02099458-0003